GERIATRICS, GERONTOLOGY AND ELDERLY ISSUES

CARE OF THE OLDER AFRICAN ADULT

Geriatrics, Gerontology and Elderly Issues

Additional books and e-books in this series can be found on Nova's website under the Series tab.

GERIATRICS, GERONTOLOGY AND ELDERLY ISSUES

CARE OF THE OLDER AFRICAN ADULT

SEKI A. BALOGUN
EDITOR

nova
Medicine & Health
New York

Library of Congress Cataloging-in-Publication Data

Names: Balogun, Seki A., editor.
Title: Care of the older African adult / Seki A. Balogun, Director, Geriatrics Fellowship Program, Associate Professor of Internal, Medicine/Physical Medicine & Rehabilitation, University of Virginia Health System, Division of General Medicine, Geriatrics and Palliative Care, Charlottesville, Virginia, USA, editor.
Description: New York : Nova Science Publishers, [2021] | Series: Geriatrics, gerontology and elderly issues | Includes bibliographical references and index. |
Identifiers: LCCN 2021009722 (print) | LCCN 2021009723 (ebook) | ISBN 9781536192957 (hardcover) | ISBN 9781536193954 (adobe pdf)
Subjects: LCSH: Geriatric nursing--Africa. | Older people--Health and hygiene--Africa.
Classification: LCC RC954 .C3713 2021 (print) | LCC RC954 (ebook) | DDC 618.97/0231--dc23
LC record available at https://lccn.loc.gov/2021009722
LC ebook record available at https://lccn.loc.gov/2021009723

Published by Nova Science Publishers, Inc. † New York

Dedicated to all of our older adult patients who
continually teach us more than they learn from us
and to all clinicians who care for geriatric-aged patients,

with love of medicine and devotion to our most vulnerable.

CONTENTS

PREFACE

Geriatric medicine is generally defined as medical care for adults aged 65 years and older. In Africa and in many developing countries, where the average life expectancy is less than 65 years, medical care of the older adult is still being defined and is in its infancy stages. There are also disparities in health and health care of older adults of African origin, in most countries across the world. The aim of this book is to provide a clinical practice resource for physicians and allied health professionals, as they deliver clinical care for older adults of African descent all over the world. It is not intended to be a comprehensive textbook for geriatric medicine, instead we focus on common health care issues and unique cultural characteristics that often impact health care utilization in this vulnerable subset of older adults. Chapter authors are medical experts from across several continents, with extensive training and experience in providing medical care for older adults of African descent.

Seki A. Balogun, MBBS, FACP, AGSF
Editor

ACKNOWLEDGMENT

Heartfelt thanks and appreciation to Mark E. Williams, MD, FACP, Professor Emeritus of Geriatric Medicine, a wonderful role model and mentor, who patiently reviewed chapters in the book and provided invaluable guidance.

In: Care of the Older African Adult
Editor: Seki A. Balogun ISBN: 978-1-53619-295-7

Chapter 1

OVERVIEW OF GERIATRIC CLINICAL CARE IN AFRICANS

Seki A. Balogun*
Associate Professor,
Internal Medicine and Geriatric Medicine,
Division of General Medicine, Geriatrics and Palliative Care,
University of Virginia Health System, Charlottesville, VA, US

ABSTRACT

The clinical care of African adults 65 years and older involves a holistic approach in treating medical issues, as well as maintaining physical, cognitive and psychosocial function. With increasing globalization, it is increasingly important for all clinicians to acquire knowledge and appropriate cultural competence in caring for older adults of widely varying societal practices and beliefs, as this facilitates better patient – physician communication, promotes trust and ultimately may improve societal health disparities. Older adults have organ specific changes that occur with normal aging and have common disorders that

* Corresponding Author's Email: sab2s@virginia.edu.

occur with advancing age, known as geriatric syndromes. Understanding, recognizing and distinguishing these age-related organ specific changes from common geriatric syndromes such as sensory impairment, falls and gait impairment, delirium, dementia, osteoporosis and urinary incontinence, is critically important in managing this vulnerable population. Knowledge of appropriate cancer screening, health maintenance recommendations and pharmacotherapy is also crucial. Furthermore, appropriate management of certain diseases such as diabetes mellitus, hypertension and prostate cancer which are more prevalent in older adults of African descent serves to maintain overall health in this subset of the population.

Keywords: geriatric care, normal aging, health maintenance, geriatric syndromes, living will, durable power of attorney for health care, physician orders for life sustaining treatment

1. Introduction

'Mrs. RT is an 80-year-old Nigerian woman with multiple medical problems including essential hypertension, chronic kidney disease stage 3, hyperlipidemia and chronic pain due to degenerative joint disease of multiple joints. She is currently in the United States visiting with her daughter for 4 months, but otherwise lives in Nigeria. She has significant limitations in ambulation and is able to walk only short distances with a front-wheeled walker within the home. She is otherwise independent of basic activities of daily living. Her daughter also notes progressive memory loss over the last year. Her medications are acetaminophen, ibuprofen, pravastatin, amlodipine, hydrochlorothiazide, multivitamin supplementation, fish oil supplement, vitamin C, vitamin D and calcium supplements. She also takes traditional herbal supplements from Nigeria for occasional diarrhea. She presents to the clinic to establish medical care.'

Geriatric Medicine, the clinical care of older adults age 65 years and older, focuses not only on the treatment of diseases, but also maintenance of health, cognitive, physical and psychosocial function. It utilizes a holistic approach, which is crucial for the care of older adults such as Mrs. RT, who often have multiple co-morbidities and require complex medical management. In providing geriatric medical care for older adults of African descent, it is important for clinicians to have appropriate cultural competence, in addition to adequate knowledge of common clinical conditions and diseases prevalent in this sub group. Cultural competence enhances awareness, knowledge and understanding of individual cultural practices and societal differences in communities all over the world. Respect for diversity in beliefs and cultural practices is a fundamental component of cultural competence. For clinicians, this lends itself to effective patient-physician communication and interactions, enabling patients to freely express themselves, promoting appropriate diagnoses, management plans and positive clinical outcomes [1, 2]. Beyond individual clinical interactions, adoption of cultural competence principles within health systems also works to promote health policies for people across all backgrounds and races, thereby reducing disparities in accessing and utilization of healthcare [3].

The African continent has great cultural diversity, made up of fifty-four countries with approximately 3000 tribes and 2000 different languages. In addition, within each country, there are very varied cultural practices and beliefs. African Americans and Africans in the diaspora also have distinct cultural practices, some of which originate from Africa while others are very different and are borne out of their ancestral experiences in their adopted countries, outside the African continent. Understanding and appreciating these cultural differences, as well as recognizing older adults of African descent as a very polylithic subgroup, are important aspects of clinical care for older African adults. Clinicians can further engender trust and foster meaningful patient- physician relationships by being open to explore individual patient's beliefs and cultural practices, particularly those beliefs that may impact health and healthcare. In this book, we explore common systemic diseases in older adults of African descent and highlight prevalent cultural practices that may impact health and healthcare utilization, across this very diverse group. This chapter provides an overview of geriatric medicine and outlines medical management of common conditions in older adults, known as geriatric syndromes, which are also discussed in detail in subsequent chapters.

2. Demography

The African population makes up about 16% of the world's total population. There are also several countries such as Brazil and United States where people of African descent make up significant proportions of the population, which are about 27% and 14% respectively. For various societal reasons, African populations also tend to be the poorest worldwide. Thirty-eight percent of the population in Africa live in extreme poverty as opposed to 0.3–7% in other continents. There are however, several African countries that have made great strides in reducing poverty levels such as Equatorial Guinea, Gabon, Mauritius and Seychelles, where the poverty levels are at less than 3% with several more countries projected to reduce poverty to the same levels by 2030. Numerous societal factors contribute to poverty on the African continent; these include poor governance, poor utilization of natural resources, prevalence of communicable diseases such as malaria and human immunodeficiency virus (HIV) infection, and historical societal exploitation by governments and external entities. With resultant lower life expectancies, African countries tend to have relatively younger populations compared to developed countries. Adults 65 years and older make up about 2-6% of the population of most African countries while the proportion of older adults in developed countries in North America and Europe is up to 16% and 20% respectively. According to the 2019 United Nations Human Development Report, the average life expectancy in many West African countries such as Nigeria is as low as 54.3 years, while in North African countries like Ethiopia and Egypt, the average life expectancy is higher at 66 years and 71.8 years respectively, which is still lower than in many developed countries in North America and Europe, where the average life expectancy ranges from 78–84.7 years.

Health disparities and lack of access to health care directly correlate with poverty level. Other factors such as low health literacy, lack of health insurance and food insecurity are also very prevalent in African communities; and are associated with the development of medical conditions such as malnutrition, diabetes mellitus and cardiac disease. Even, in many developed countries such as the United States, the median household income is the lowest in black communities. These factors often contribute to poor health outcomes in older adults of African descent both on the African continent and in many developed countries [4].

3. Normal Aging

Normal aging is a progressive physiological process that affects all organ systems. It is heterogeneous, with a highly variable rate of aging that is specific to individuals. The aging process is significantly affected by genetic characteristics, environmental factors and lifestyle preferences. These age-associated changes tend to decrease the functional organ reserves making it difficult for the older body to maintain homeostasis and thereby leading to increased susceptibility to disease development or pathology.

Frailty is often at the latter point of aging, where physiologic and functional reserves are maximally utilized such that any additional insult or injury such as an infection or trauma, predispose to systemic or organ-specific decompensation. This decompensation presents in many ways in older adults, including delirium, functional decline or worsening of organic function such as heart failure and kidney disease. Organ systems such as cardiovascular, renal, genitourinary and central nervous system are affected to a greater degree with normal aging. Often times, it is difficult to differentiate from these changes from pathological diseases, especially when there are concomitant chronic medical conditions. Organ specific physiologic changes associated with normal aging are outlined.

The aging central nervous system is characterized by decreased brain volume with reduced cerebral blood flow and loss of neurons. Neurofibrillary tangles and senile plaques are also seen with normal aging but much less than with Alzheimer's dementia. There are also age- related changes in brain neurotransmitter and receptors. Functionally, the normal aging brain is cognitively intact with preserved remote memory. However, there is some slowing of brain processing speed, particularly after the sixth decade, which may mildly affect executive function and performance on timed cognitive testing but does not significantly affect the ability to engage in basic or instrumental activities of daily living, which are essential daily activities that older adults require to be able to successfully live independently in their homes and communities. Mild cognitive impairment (MCI) and Dementia are not considered to be physiological or part of the normal aging process. Both are associated with decreased ability to perform activities of daily living.

The cardiovascular system develops modest anatomic changes with mild left atrial enlargement and left ventricular hypertrophy with aging. There is also aortic and mitral valve thickening and calcification which predispose to heart conduction problems. With normal aging, there is also increased large artery stiffness which is amplified with diseases such as hypertension. The risks for comorbid hypertension and coronary artery disease are increased with aging, in conjunction with lifestyle factors such as decreased physical activity. Exercise has been found to attenuate these age-associated cardiac effects.

With the respiratory system, anatomic and functional changes make aging lungs susceptible to pneumonia and hypoxia. Enlargement of alveolar ducts due to loss of elastic tissue and alterations in collagen fibers lead to decreased surface area for gas exchange and increased anatomic pulmonary dead space. Aging lungs are also predisposed to atelectasis due to increased chest wall stiffness with resultant reduced lung compliance. This, coupled with reduced mucociliary clearance, makes recovery from a pulmonary insult like an infection much slower in older adults.

The renal system is significantly affected by aging with progressive reduction in renal mass starting as early as age 30 years. Atrophy of nephrons and glomeruli sclerosis contribute to decrease in kidney function with aging, affecting creatinine clearance to very variable degrees. In a 1990 cross sectional study of healthy older adults, only one third had significant decline in glomerular filtration rate (GFR), while two thirds had slight or no change in GFR [5]. In stressful conditions such as decreased hydration, these changes also impair the ability of the aging kidney to maintain appropriate fluid and electrolyte balance. In addition, older adults are more prone to nephrotoxicity from certain medications or intravenous contrast and the resultant kidney injury is more often longer lasting compared to the younger population.

The gastrointestinal system has modest anatomic changes with aging. Thinning of epithelial layers of oral mucosa and decrease in saliva production predispose to dry mouth with resultant tooth decay and difficulty with adequate mastication of food. These, ultimately may affect nutritional status. Certain medications such as anticholinergics, also contribute to dry mouth in many older adults. In addition, there is mucosal and villus atrophy throughout the GI tract with minimal reduction in absorption of nutrients and dysmotility predisposing to constipation in older adults.

Liver function declines with decrease in liver perfusion and mass, though liver enzyme values on standard tests are minimally affected with aging. Liver functions such as metabolic clearance of medications involving cytochrome P450 and synthesis of vitamin K dependent clotting factors are reduced leading to longer half-life of drugs and increased susceptibility of older adults to medications such as warfarin.

The hematologic system is also modestly affected with aging. There is overall normal function throughout a person's lifespan, however there is reduced functional reserve with increased fatty infiltration in bone marrow with aging, so compensatory response to insults like bleeding is delayed and stunted. Platelet responsiveness and levels of some clotting factors also increase, predisposing to a procoagulant state and increased risk for deep venous thrombosis in older individuals with functional decline.

With aging, the genitourinary system undergoes anatomic and functional changes which include decrease in detrusor muscle contractility, bladder capacity and ability to withhold urination due to decreased innervation of detrusor muscle, leading to increased risk of urinary incontinence. This tends to be more common in women than men up until after age 80 years, at which point the prevalence is similar in both genders. In older men, enlargement of the prostate contributes to urinary incontinence, as a result of poor urinary stream and urinary retention with elevated post void residual bladder volume. There also tends to be reduced sexual activity, particularly after age 80 years with associated decline in reproductive function as a result of reduction in sperm production, impaired sperm motility and increased chromosomal abnormality. With older menopausal women, there is vaginal atrophy and dryness from loss of estrogen. This leads to dyspareunia and elevation in vaginal pH, leading to increased bacterial colonization and predisposition to urinary tract infections.

The musculoskeletal system is characterized by loss of muscle mass with atrophy and denervation of muscle fibers, in addition to fatty infiltration of muscle. This process known as sarcopenia, is associated with decreased muscle strength and function. It occurs at different rates in older adults and generally accelerates with aging. There is also delayed healing after muscle injury in older adults due to decreased ability of muscle cells to regenerate. Hormonal variation also contributes to these muscle changes as people age. These hormonal changes also affect bone mass and predispose to osteoporosis particularly in postmenopausal women.

The skin with normal aging undergoes atrophy and decreased elasticity. These changes increase skin sagging, wrinkling and skin fragility leading to easy bruising and skin tears from mild shear stress. Vitamin D synthesis which is crucial for bone health, occurs in the epidermis through conversion of 7-hydrocholesterol to pre-vitamin D3 and is also adversely affected in normal aging.

With the sensory system, the eyes, ears, sense of taste and smell are all affected with normal aging. Structural age-related changes lead to periorbital tissue atrophy and eyelid laxity with resultant ectropion or entropion. Presbyopia gradually develops by the fourth decade due to decreased lens and iris elasticity, making it difficult for older adults to focus on near objects. Presbycusis, high-frequency hearing loss occurs due to age-related structural changes in the middle and inner ear, and is associated with difficulty with speech discrimination, particularly in a noisy environment. The sense of smell also decreases with normal aging, largely due to loss of olfactory neurons, this in turn adversely affects the sense of taste.

Normal aging also affects the immune responses making older adults more susceptible to infections, autoimmune disorders and certain malignancies.

4. Health Maintenance

Maintaining good health hinges on the prevention or control of illnesses before symptoms occur that may affect the quantity and/or quality of life. The health and wellbeing of older adults are dependent on several factors, including the aging process, functional ability and social health determinants which vary widely in African communities worldwide. Clinicians providing care for these older adults, therefore need to consider not only individual needs but also societal factors. For instance, it may be appropriate to focus on certain cancer screening tests for a 70 year old black woman living in the United States with greater access to imaging tests compared to a 70 year old black woman living in certain parts of sub-Saharan Africa, where the preventative focus may need to be more on immunizations against infections and other screening tests that are more accessible. It is also prudent for clinicians of older adults of African descent to explore individual cultural beliefs and practices that may impact attitudes towards health maintenance, particularly in regards to preventative testing and immunization. In many African cultures, people seek medical care out of necessity, often when sick and after trying alternative medicines such as herbs and traditional concoctions. So, the concept of health maintenance through preventative testing, when one is well, may be viewed as foreign and un-necessary. While in some African American communities, there is still great mistrust of the medical system borne out of a history of racist medical practices where African Americans where unfavorably treated and in many cases, exploited. For clinicians, it is important to be aware of some of these cultural differences and to thoughtfully explore these views as they provide medical care for older African adults, while also recognizing how widely varying these beliefs are, from one community to another.

In assessing the individual preventative health care needs of older adults, several factors that impact estimated average life expectancy need to be considered as well, and should not be based solely on the patient's age. Many preventative test guidelines utilize age limits based on average life expectancy calculations which in addition to age, also consider factors such as country of residence, physical function and presence of chronic diseases. It is also important to critically analyze the risks and benefits of preventative tests in relation to the individual under consideration, making sure that the benefits of the test overweigh the relative risks. In addition, individual preferences and goals for medical care should be considered. Screening and prevention of common medical conditions in older adults involve the following: general lifestyle recommendations, screening for cardiovascular diseases and diabetes mellitus, immunizations, screening for common cancers and evaluation for common geriatric conditions also known as geriatric syndromes. Older adults are uniquely predisposed and highly susceptible to these geriatric syndromes, mainly as a result of the aging process. Common geriatric syndromes include: osteoporosis, sensory impairment (vision and hearing), falls and gait impairment, malnutrition, urinary incontinence, dementia, delirium and osteoporosis.

4.1. General Lifestyle Recommendations

Adopting a healthy lifestyle is crucial for older adults as it promotes general wellbeing and reduces disability risk. Adequate physical activity is important, with health benefits at all ages including the frailest older adults [6]. Physical activity guidelines from the American Heart Association (AHA) and the American College of Sport Medicine (ACSM) for adults over 65 years recommend a minimum of 30 minutes of moderate intensity aerobic exercises, five days per week or a minimum of 20 minutes of vigorous intensity activity, three days per week. Muscle strengthening, flexibility and balance exercises such as Tai Chi are also recommended to maintain gait stability and prevent falls. It is important to introduce these exercises as individualized, relatable plans with gradual advancement and careful consideration of the person's baseline physical function and co-morbid chronic medical conditions, so as to avoid injury and foster adherence [7]. For instance, encouraging exercises to which the patient is already familiar is likely to yield better compliance as opposed to trying to introduce an exercise regimen that is completely new. Also, recommending simple exercises such as walking, particularly for those patients with more sedentary lifestyles, has a higher probability of being well received.

Evaluating older adults for lifestyle choices such as tobacco and alcohol use is also very important. Specific questions on the frequency and quantity of alcohol and tobacco use are recommended. Older persons can be screened for alcohol abuse or dependence using the CAGE questionnaire which is made of 4 questions and is a quick screening tool that can be utilized in the clinical setting: have you ever felt you should *Cut down* on your drinking?, have people *Annoyed* you by criticizing your drinking?, have you ever felt bad or *Guilty* about your drinking?, and have you ever taken a drink first thing in the morning *(Eye-opener)* to steady your nerves or get rid of a hangover? [8]. Confirming at least one of the questions suggests alcohol abuse or dependence. Regular counseling for smoking cessation and reduction in alcohol intake is recommended. Other options for smoking cessation in older adults include nicotine replacement therapies or medications such as bupropion or varenicline. It is also important to involve local community social support services for substance abuse when needed and available, as this fosters trust and acceptance.

4.2. Screening for Cardiovascular Diseases and Diabetes Mellitus

There is a high prevalence of hypertension and diabetes mellitus in older adults, especially in older black adults, with higher prevalence rates compared their white counterparts. These disparities are also seen in rural vs. urban older populations in communities worldwide, including Africa. Some of these disparities could be as a result of health care accessibility and utilization in these communities [9]. Screening and management of cardiovascular diseases and diabetes are discussed in detail in subsequent chapters on cardiac diseases and endocrine diseases respectively.

4.3. Immunizations

Vaccines for specific diseases are recommended in older adults. The United States Centers for Disease Control and Prevention, and Advisory Committee on Immunization Practices recommend the following vaccinations for older adults 65 years and older.

- *Tetanus vaccine:* Booster vaccines are recommended of tetanus with diphtheria toxoid (Td) or tetanus with pertussis (Tdap) vaccine every ten years. This is especially important in Africa and South America where these diseases are more prevalent. Tdap is also of great importance for older adults, such as grandparents or child care providers, who are in close contact with children younger than a year old, because of the susceptibility of children to pertussis.
- *Influenza Vaccine*: It is recommended that all adults receive influenza vaccine yearly. This is especially important in older adults as they have disproportionately high morbidity and mortality from influenza respiratory infections.
- *Pneumococcal Vaccine:* Pneumococcal pneumonia is highly prevalent in older adults and is associated with high mortality and morbidity, particularly after age 65 years. The current recommendation is that all adults receive a one-time dose of 23-valent polysaccharide pneumococcal vaccine (PPSV23) at age 65 years. For immunocompromised, high risk older adults such as those with asplenia or human immunodeficiency virus infection, PPSV23 revaccination is recommended every five to ten years. The 13-valent pneumococcal conjugate vaccine (PCV13) may also be given to high risk, immunocompromised older adults but is not currently recommended for the general older population

- *Herpes zoster vaccine:* Herpes zoster also known as shingles results from a reactivation of latent varicella zoster virus and usually results in a painful dermatomal rash. Herpes zoster is common and affects about 30 percent of adults over a lifetime with significantly increased incidence and morbidity in late life, as well as complications such as postherpetic neuralgia and encephalitis. The recombinant adjuvant zoster vaccine has a higher efficacy compared to the live attenuated zoster vaccine preparation and the current recommendation is for 2 doses of the recombinant adjuvant zoster vaccine starting at age 50 years, 2 -6 months apart [10].

4.4. Cancer Screening

In approaching cancer screening in older adults, it is important to consider the risks and benefits of the screening test. Often times the risks are immediate and usually related to the screening procedure while the benefits are long term, in many cases, up to 10 years. Therefore, screening for cancers in older adults is most beneficial in those with estimated life expectancy of 10 years or more. Other factors such as co-morbid conditions and baseline health need to be explored in cancer screening discussions, as well as personal preferences, cultural beliefs and values. Clinicians facilitate this through a supportive, shared decision-making process. It is again crucial to bear in mind that in some African cultures or communities, the concept of preventive medical care may be considered foreign and therefore screening tests in an asymptomatic person, particularly those that are invasive may be viewed with skepticism and reluctance. Careful consideration of these beliefs and education on the importance of screening tests are crucial in these situations. Discussing when to stop cancer screening is also important in the care of older adults and may be difficult for some who are accustomed to more aggressive therapeutic options and may view this unfavorably or as ageist. While for others, it may be a relief not to have to bother with additional tests, particularly if invasive. Most cancer screening clinical guidelines do not recommend screening beyond age 75 years and for some older adults with multiple co-morbidities and estimated life expectancy less than 10 years, the risks of screening may overweigh the expected long-term benefits. In such patients, the need for continued cancer screening and possible consideration of stopping screening may need to be explored before age 75 years. At the same time, otherwise healthy older patients at moderate to high risk for cancer, with minimal co-morbidities, intact physical and cognitive function may opt to continue cancer screening well into advanced ages. Screening recommendations are mainly for cancers in which early detection and subsequent treatment make a significant difference in morbidity and mortality. The screening test which may be invasive, needs to be safe with minimal procedural risks.

Screening tests for common cancers are discussed below.

4.4.1. Breast Cancer

Mammogram is the preferred screening test for breast cancer and is typically recommended every one to two years for women with average risk, between ages 50 to 74 years, depending on preference. Screening mammograms have a mortality risk reduction benefit of 14-33% in this age group [11]. For women with high risk of breast cancer such as those with a personal or significant family history of breast cancer, consideration should be given to starting screening much earlier than 50 years and later than 74 years, depending on the person's co-morbidities, preference, functional and cognitive status.

4.4.2. Prostate Cancer

Current recommendations for prostate cancer screening involve discussions of the risks and benefits of screening in men age 50–69 years. Special consideration should be given to men with higher risk of prostate cancer such as black men, those with a history of prostate cancer in a first degree relative or genetic mutation. Screening is dependent on the patient's preference, risk factors for prostate cancer and life expectancy; and is typically done with obtaining prostate specific antigen level [12].

4.4.3. Colorectal Cancer

Colorectal screening is recommended between ages 50–75 years for average risk adults. There is also some evidence to support starting screening at age 45 years, in certain demographic groups with a higher incidence of colorectal cancer, such as in the black population. The decision and choice of colorectal screening test is dependent on the presence of comorbidities, life expectancy of 10 or more years, patient's preference and test availability. Some of the colorectal tests are non-invasive (such as the fecal immunochemical test and guaiac-based fecal occult blood), and convenient but require frequent yearly testing. Multitarget stool DNA testing is also non-invasive, convenient and in addition, has a higher sensitivity for detecting colorectal cancer. This is recommended every 3 years. Colorectal tests such as colonoscopy and flexible sigmoidoscopy are invasive, require extensive bowel preparation prior to procedure, which can be quite taxing for many older adults, but retesting is recommended every 5–10 years, depending on risk factors such as personal or family history of colorectal cancer. Colonoscopy has the highest sensitivity of all the screening tests for colorectal cancer, however it is the most invasive and carries higher procedural risks. As such, special consideration of patients' comorbidities, functional status and average life expectancy must be undertaken when exploring which of these modalities would offer the most benefit with minimal risk. In addition, the availability of these tests are very variable in different communities with limitations due to cost and availability of health care professionals. This, invariably would also affect test choice.

4.4.4. Cervical Cancer

Cervical cancer screening is performed with Pap smear. Recommendations are to discontinue screening at age 65 years in those with low to average risk of cervical cancer, provided there have been three consecutive negative cytology tests within the last ten years and the most recent at least five years prior to discontinuation. Two prior consecutive negative human papillomavirus/pap co-tests are also considered adequate cervical cancer screening and subsequent screening can be discontinued in that situation. Women who have had hysterectomy due to a non-cancerous pathology do not require pap smears. Older adults at higher risk for cervical cancer such as those with prior cervical cancer, new sexual partner or smokers may need continued screening beyond age 65 years, if their functional status is intact and life expectancy is 10 years or more.

4.4.5. Lung Cancer

The United States Preventative Services Task Force recommends yearly low-dose CT scan screening for lung cancer in high-risk individuals ages 55 to 80 years with a 30 pack-year history of smoking and who are either current smokers or quit within past 15 years. In a 2011 study, screening with low CT scan in these high-risk individuals resulted in a lung cancer related mortality reduction of 20% [13]. The availability and cost of the test is a significant limitation for many communities and countries worldwide, particularly in Africa. Discontinuation of screening is recommended with limited life expectancy or when smoking cessation has been for 15 years or more.

5. Geriatric Syndromes

5.1. Sensory Impairment: Vision and Hearing

Visual impairment is very common in older adults with a prevalence of 4–24% in adults 50 years and older worldwide. Older adults in Africa and South Asia are affected to a higher degree than those in more developed countries in Europe and North America [14]. Age associated changes in vision often leads to presbyopia, a non-refractive disorder in which the lens loses its power of accommodation. The aging eye is also susceptible to several pathologic processes which are leading causes of visual impairment worldwide. The most common of which are cataracts, glaucoma and macular degeneration. The high prevalence of chronic diseases such as hypertension and diabetes mellitus also predispose older adults to these ocular disorders. Often times, the loss of vision in older adults is associated with falls, decline in overall health with cognitive and physical functional decline resulting in significant impairment in activities of daily living. With geriatric assessments, it is important to include specific questions about vision, in addition to eye examination and vision screening when eye disorders are suspected. Prompt referral to ophthalmology is also critical to prevent further morbidity from loss of vision. Routine vision screening for asymptomatic, low risk older adults without any comorbidities is generally not recommended as there is insufficient evidence that it significantly improves outcomes.

With regards to hearing loss from presbycusis, a World Health Organization 2012 report estimates that about a third of adults 65 years and older worldwide have significant hearing loss, with the highest prevalence in sub-Saharan Africa and South Asia. It is often associated with low self-esteem, social isolation with resultant depression and decline in overall function. Inquiry about hearing loss is also important, as part of a thorough geriatric assessment. Prompt referral for pure audiometry, which is the gold standard for detection of suspected hearing loss, is important to improve quality of life and the associated morbidity.

5.2. Falls and Gait Impairment

Falls in older adults are very common and are the leading cause of injury in this population subset with associated significant morbidity and mortality [15]. Falls are a major threat to the independence of older adults and tend to occur more often in those 85 years and older. Injuries with falls may result in decline physical function and overall health, in addition to possibly leading to long term care placement. Trauma from falls range from minor soft tissue bruises to major injuries such as lacerations, head trauma and fractures. Though a small percentage of falls directly result in death, fall complications are the leading cause of death from injury in older adults [16].

In addition to advanced age, risk factors for falling include history of prior falls, presence of cognitive or physical impairment, gait imbalance, use of medications such as antihypertensives, sedatives, psychotropics, and presence of orthostatic hypotension [17]. Presence of chronic medical conditions that affect cognitive or functional impairment also predispose to falls. These include Parkinson's disease, diabetes mellitus, stroke and rheumatologic joint diseases.

With clinical evaluation of older adults, an assessment for risk of falls should incorporated at least yearly, as older adults may not report this to their clinicians. A multifactorial falls risk assessment includes taking a comprehensive history of prior falls, medication or substance use history and reviewing chronic medical conditions. Physical examination should include a gait assessment, test for function and balance, all of which may be useful in identifying older adults at high risk for falls. Functional tests include the 'Get up and Go' test which involves having the patient get up from a standard chair, walk a fixed distance of about 10 feet (3 meters), walk back and sit down. The examiner observes the patient's gait, balance and ease of getting up during these movements. Timed variations of the test have been used to some degree to further delineate those at higher risk of falls [18]. Other tests for gait and balance include the performance-oriented mobility assessment and berg balance test. These measure functional ability in sitting, standing, transfers, and a careful gait and balance assessment.

Physical examination should also include assessment for orthostatic hypotension, tests for visual acuity and vestibular function. Neurologic and lower extremity examinations including motor and sensory function, in addition to assessment for possible joint deformities are also very important. Laboratory testing should be tailored to chronic medical conditions and identified risk factors.

In managing older adults with falls, a multidisciplinary approach has been found to be most effective. This typically involves physical therapy referral for exercises focused on gait, balance and strength training, in addition to home safety evaluation through occupational therapy. Some older adults may require the use of assistive gait devices to aid safe ambulation. A review of medications is also important, to identify those that may increase the risk for falls such as sedatives and anticholinergic medications. Managing comorbidities and other fall risk factors such as visual impairment, orthostatic hypotension, joint deformities, are also critical aspects of care. These multifactorial interventions are important in falls prevention as well. Other interventions such as the use of hip protectors have limited utility due to poor compliance from discomfort when worn. Screening and treatment of osteoporosis is also considered part of falls management as this potentially reduces the risk of hip fractures [19].

5.3. Malnutrition

Malnutrition encompasses undernutrition and overnutrition. Undernutrition is commonly defined as body mass index (BMI) less than 18.5. BMI between 18.5 and 24.9 are generally considered normal. Overnutrition includes overweight (BMI between 25 and 29.9) and obesity (BMI 30 and above). It is important to note that while these are generally acceptable BMI ranges for all races, there is great racial variability in body build, with blacks generally tending to have more of a heavy, muscular build compared to Caucasians and Asians, with some differences in relative body fat content. Individual BMI levels should therefore be considered in this context when providing medical care for older black adults [20].

Undernutrition is more prevalent in older adults than overnutrition and is associated with increased mortality [21]. There is also an increased risk of sarcopenia and resultant decline in physical function with undernutrition in older adults, particularly with inadequate protein intake [22]. Worldwide, the prevalence of malnutrition is between 1-15% in ambulatory older adults in ambulatory settings, with up to 50% of older adults at risk for developing malnutrition. In older adults in long term care institutions and those acutely hospitalized, the prevalence of malnutrition is much higher and is up to 65% in many countries in Europe, United States and South Africa [23, 24]. Risk factors for inadequate nutrition include socioeconomic issues, food insecurity, presence of chronic medical comorbidities that adversely affect swallowing and appetite such as depression, anxiety, Parkinson's disease, dementia, diabetes mellitus, malignancy and stroke. Dental issues and age related decline in taste and smell also affect oral food intake. For some older adults, cognitive and functional impairments may limit their access and ability to prepare nutritious meals. In these cases, the presence of adequate social support and feeding assistance is crucial.

In geriatric clinical assessments, an evaluation of nutritional status is important. This can usually be done through enquiring about diet and caloric intake. It is also important to specifically ask about any change in dietary habits. Serial weight measurements also provide useful information. Unintentional weight loss of at least 5% in 3 months or 10% in 6 months are considered clinically significant and should prompt further evaluation to identify contributory factors for undernutrition [25]. A complete physical examination including an oral assessment is important. Initial laboratory tests for biochemical and inflammatory conditions such as complete blood count, basic metabolic panel, glucose and thyroid function are usually warranted. Additional clinical work up would depend on potential etiologies identified during clinical assessment. These may include chest imaging for possible pulmonary infections such as tuberculosis, which may be associated with weight loss and is prevalent in many countries worldwide. Other possible tests are swallowing studies and endoscopy for esophageal pathologies and inflammatory markers such as C-reactive protein, which is found in cachexia related to malignancy and chronic infections.

Managing undernutrition in older adults involves treatment of underlying etiologies such as depression and ensuring adequate caloric intake. As part of the effort to increase caloric intake, dietary restrictions such as those with diabetes, may need to be eliminated and foods that appeal to the specific individual encouraged. It is also important to consider regional and ethnic food preferences. Consultation with a dietician may also be necessary to ensure adequate and appropriate dietary options. In addition, providing feeding assistance to those with significant cognitive and functional impairment is crucial. Protein nutritional supplements may have some utility in undernourished older adults in acute hospital and long-term care settings, including home care [26].

Mirtazapine, an atypical antidepressant that indirectly increases the release of norepinephrine and serotonin, is commonly used as an appetite stimulant in patients with weight loss related to depression. A few studies on mirtazapine have shown weight gain benefit in older adults with weight loss, particularly those with dementia [27]. It also tends to be well tolerated in older adults, particularly at lower doses.

Other appetite stimulants such as megestrol and dronabinol have some utility in patients with cachexia related to cancer or acquired immunodeficiency syndrome (AIDS), with modest weight gain and increase in appetite. Both have limited utility in older adults and are associated with several adverse effects. Megestrol is associated with edema, deep venous thrombosis and increased mortality in older adults in long term care [28, 29], while dronabinol has significant central nervous system side effects such as cognitive impairment, seizures, hallucinations and depression. Growth hormone secretagogues (GHS) have shown some promise in studies, in stimulating appetite and increase lean muscle mass but there is limited data with older adults with weight loss or cachexia [30]. GHS are also associated with adverse effects such as hyperglycemia and nausea. These appetite stimulants are usually not recommended in older adults.

Overnutrition in older adults tends to be associated with less mortality risks compared to younger age groups, though there are risks of increased disability in overweight or obese older adults. Weight loss in these older adults have similar benefits in physical function and quality of life as seen in younger adults, particularly with comorbid chronic medical conditions such as osteoarthritis, obstructive sleep apnea and diabetes mellitus [31]. As with all age groups, regular exercise and dietary modification are the mainstay of treatment for obesity. In older adults, dietary modification with high protein content tends to decrease risk of sarcopenia by preserving muscle mass and function, while leading to weight loss.

Micronutrient deficiencies are also common in older adults. The most common deficiencies are vitamin D, vitamin B12 and calcium. Vitamin D deficiency is common in older adults due to age-related skin related changes with decreased synthesis of pre-vitamin D, decreased sun exposure and decreased oral vitamin D intake. Older black adults are more prone to vitamin D deficiency due to decreased skin production of pre-vitamin D. Normal 25- hydroxyvitamin D level is 30 ng/mL and above. Low vitamin levels are associated with functional decline, muscle weakness, risk of falls and fractures. Vitamin D supplementation, usually in the form of cholecalciferol (vitamin D3), is recommended for all older adults for optimal bone and muscle health, at doses of 600 – 800 Units daily. Dietary sources high in vitamin D are also advised. For older adults with low vitamin D level, high doses of oral supplementation either in the form of vitamin D3 or ergocalciferol (vitamin D2) is often warranted. Periodic monitoring of 25-hydroxyvitamin D about 3 -4 months is recommended during supplementation to avoid vitamin D toxicity.

Inadequate calcium intake and decreased gastrointestinal absorption of calcium occur with advancing age. Calcium, in addition to vitamin D are vital nutrients for bone health and critical to osteoporosis prevention and treatment. Dietary recommendation for calcium in diet and supplementation for older adults is 1200mg/day. Foods rich in calcium are generally preferred to calcium supplementation when available.

Vitamin B12 deficiency in older adults, is thought to be due to poor gastric absorption from intrinsic factor deficiency. Older adults with vitamin B12 deficiency may develop macrocytic anemia and neuropsychologic symptoms such as paresthesia, numbness of extremities, memory deficits, mood changes and psychosis. Older adults with macrocytosis and/or suggestive symptoms should be screened for vitamin B12 deficiency through vitamin B12 assays. Borderline low serum vitamin B12 levels require follow up measurement of serum methylmalonic acid, a metabolite of vitamin B12 which confirms the diagnosis, if elevated. Oral or parenteral vitamin B12 supplementation is the main stay of treatment. Also, encouraging adequate vitamin B12 in diet is recommended.

Use of multivitamins in older adults is generally recommended for those with inadequate oral intake with the aim of supplementing micronutrients in the diet.

5.4. Urinary Incontinence

Urinary incontinence (UI) is common in older adults and is a cause of significant emotional distress with social and functional implications. Urinary incontinence is often viewed as a social stigma and an embarrassment, making it difficult for those affected to socially interact with others and limiting activities of daily living. For caregivers of older adults, it is often one of the more difficult aspects of care and is a major factor in long term care placement. The prevalence of UI in independent older adults ranges from 2 to 55 percent, with higher prevalence in women and older adults in long term institutions [32, 33].

Specifically inquiring about urinary incontinence in geriatric assessments is important as many patients may not voluntarily raise this as a concern for a variety of reasons. Some may view this as part of normal aging and others may be embarrassed. Appropriate history and physical examination may be able to determine the chronicity, associated symptoms and the type of incontinence such as stress, overflow, urge or mixed incontinence. Laboratory testing such as urinalysis, complete blood counts, electrolytes are usually recommended to assess for infections, metabolic disorders such as diabetes and kidney dysfunction. Treatments can usually be tailored to the type of incontinence with varying levels of effectivity. Referral to a urologist or urogynecologist (for women) may also be warranted. This is discussed in detail in the chapter on urogynecologic diseases.

5.5. Dementia/Delirium

Dementia and Delirium are neurological conditions that occur almost exclusively in older adults. Dementia refers to a chronic and permanent decline in multiple domains of cognitive abilities with significant impairment in activities of daily living. It encompasses all types of dementia including Alzheimer's disease, vascular dementia, dementia with lewy bodies and frontotemporal dementia. Delirium is an acute and usually temporary change in cognition characterized by inattention, with an underlying precipitating medical condition or adverse effect from medications. Both dementia and delirium may affect different domains of cognition including memory, language, visuospatial function and perception. Dementia tends to be progressive over months to years while with delirium, there may be daily fluctuations in cognitive abilities which typically last days to weeks and improve with treatment of underlying medical condition or removal of offending medication. There may also neuropsychiatric symptoms in both conditions such as mood disturbances, behavioral changes, agitation, delusions and hallucinations, which tend to be mostly visual.

Delirium is common, particularly in older hospitalized adults and those with baseline cognitive impairment. Prevalence is up to 40 percent, particularly with complex surgeries such as neurosurgery, hip fracture surgery or cardiac surgery [34]. Other precipitating factors include anticholinergic or psychoactive medications, polypharmacy, infections, dehydration, immobility, malnutrition and iatrogenic measures such as indwelling bladder catheters. Dementia is also increasingly common with older age groups. Alzheimer's Dementia occurs in up to 60 per 1000 older adults [35]. Other dementias such as vascular dementia and dementia with lewy body occur to a lesser degree.

In clinical situations, delirium and dementia may have similar presentations. Often times, older adults with underlying dementia may develop delirium, which may further complicate the clinical picture. A detailed history and physical examination is important to help with differentiating between the two conditions. Often times, the caregivers' input is crucial in being able to get an accurate account of the patient's illness and chronology of symptoms. A detailed medication review is also very important.

Treatment of delirium mainly consists of treating underlying medical condition or removing high risk medications, while the treatment of dementia varies widely depending on the type of dementia. With Alzheimer's Dementia, the main components of therapy are supportive care, behavioral therapies and pharmacotherapy with acetylcholinesterase inhibitors such as donepezil, galantamine, rivastigmine and memantine, an N-methyl-D-aspartate receptor antagonist and dopamine agonist. With other types of dementias such as vascular dementia, managing risk factors for cardiovascular disease such as hypertension, hyperlipidemia, diabetes mellitus and atrial fibrillation, is of vital importance. This is further discussed in detail in the chapter on neuropsychiatric disorders.

5.6. Osteoporosis

Osteoporosis is a bone metabolic disorder defined by decreased bone mass with structural defects leading to bone fragility and fractures. The World Health Organization's definition of osteoporosis is based on comparison of the bone mineral density to the reference mean bone mineral density of young female adults (T-score). A bone mineral density consistent with a T- score of less than or equal to 2.5 standard deviations below the reference mean meets the criterion for osteoporosis [36]. Postmenopausal women and older men are predisposed to osteoporosis, as a result of changes in bone metabolism related to aging. Other risk factors include low body weight, poor nutrition, tobacco use and family history of osteoporosis. Adults with African ancestry and those with higher BMI tend to have slower bone loss with aging and therefore a lower incidence of osteoporosis. In geriatric assessments, it is important to specifically enquire about risk factors for osteoporosis and history of prior fractures. A dual energy x-ray absorptiometry (DEXA) is typically utilized to assess bone density and is the diagnostic gold standard for osteoporosis. Other modalities such as heel ultrasound, provide a peripheral measurement of bone density, tend to be cheaper and more readily available for use in osteoporosis screening. However, this provides much lower correlation with hip and spine bone mass, which are the primary sites of major osteoporotic fractures.

Optimal nutrition with adequate calcium, vitamin D intake and regular exercise are critical in osteoporosis treatment. In addition, pharmacotherapy with bisphosphonates may be considered for those at high risk of fractures. Anabolic agents such as parathyroid hormone analogs are usually not used as first line agents but may be considered if there is an intolerance to bisphosphonates or in cases of severe osteoporosis. Osteoporosis is discussed in detail in the chapter on endocrine disorders.

6. PHARMACOTHERAPY

Older adults are generally prescribed the highest proportion of medications. In the United States (US), those 65 years and older make up about 12% of population yet a third of all physician prescriptions are given to this subset of the population. By the year 2040, it is expected that adults 65 years and older will grow to about a quarter of the general US population and take up to half of all prescribed medications. Polypharmacy is also very common in older adults with up to 30% of older adults taking at least five prescribed medications and about 12% taking ten or more medications. The highest rate of medication use is in those age 75–85 years, with up to half of these older adults taking concurrent 'over the counter' (non-prescribed) medications, dietary supplements and herbal medications [37, 38]. This is also very prevalent in older African adults, particularly the concurrent use of herbal remedies which may have interactions with prescribed medications. The reasons for polypharmacy include the presence of high chronic disease burden in older adults often leading to multiple physician visits and prescribers. In rural populations, lower educational level may also be a contributory factor. Polypharmacy places these older adults at increased risk for adverse drug effects either from drug-drug interactions or drug-disease interactions, and are a major cause of morbidity and mortality associated with emergent hospitalizations in many instances [39]. In a 2018 study of older South African adults, the prevalence of serious adverse drug effects was about 26% [40]. With polypharmacy, there is also the increased likelihood of reduced medication compliance as older adults will often have difficulty with complex medication regimens, particularly if there is cognitive or functional impairment.

In addition to factors above, older adults are at increased risk for adverse drug effects from physiologic changes that occur as a result of normal aging which affect the different pharmacokinetic phases to varying degrees. Drug metabolism and elimination phases are most significantly affected due to age related changes in liver and kidney function respectively. These mostly lead to reduced clearance of medications leading to prolongation of their effect. The distribution phase of drug pharmacokinetics in older adults is also affected due to relative decrease in lean muscle mass and body water, with greater fat stores. This leads to higher volumes of distribution for those medications that are fat soluble compared to water soluble medications. This also contributes to prolonged effect of fat soluble medications such as benzodiazepines, antidepressants and antipsychotics. The pharmokinetic process of certain medications such as warfarin and digoxin that bind to plasma proteins, is also affected with resultant higher proportion of unbound and pharmacologically active metabolites of these drugs in older adults compared to younger adults, from age-related decrease in lean muscle mass and plasma proteins. In such medications, care must be taken to administer appropriately dose – adjusted drug amounts and monitor the free portion of these drug levels, when possible.

With all the age-related pharmacokinetic and pharmacodynamic changes, potentially inappropriate medications (PIMs) in older adults have been clearly defined. The American Geriatrics Society (AGS) Beers Criteria is a widely used clinical tool which identifies common PIMs in different medication groups such as anticholinergic medications, cardiovascular medications (alpha-1 blockers, central alpha agonists, antiarrhythmics), benzodiazepines and antipsychotics, which are associated with significant adverse drug events in older adults [41]. The AGS Beers criteria has also been used as an indicator of quality clinical care of older adults, particularly in long term care settings, as well as in many clinical studies. The use of PIMs is prevalent in older adults worldwide. In a recent study of South African older adults, about 68 percent had at least one PIM, while another study in Brazilian older adults, the prevalence was about 42 percent [42, 43].

In providing care for older adults, clinicians should review their medication regimens with every clinical encounter, including inquiries about any non-prescribed ('over the counter') medications, herbal remedies and supplements. In some instances, it may be prudent to have the patient bring in all of medications to the clinical encounter, so a detailed medication reconciliation is performed. It is also important for clinicians to continually try to simplify medication regimens either by eliminating any unnecessary medications or limiting the number of medications prescribed, when possible. It may be advisable in some clinical conditions, to consider non-pharmacological therapies first before prescribing systemic medications. For instance, with osteoarthritis, one may prescribe topical analgesia and physical therapy first before considering oral analgesics. In addition, medication regimens should be carefully examined for PIMs, drug-drug interactions and appropriate medication dosing as some drugs may need to be adjusted for kidney function. In starting a medication in older adults, the lowest possible dose is often recommended with gradual titration as indicated. Geriatricians often describe this process with the phrase – 'start low, go slow.' With some frail older adults, half of the normal adult starting dose may be appropriate, particularly if they have a low body mass index. Careful observation with any new medication regimen is also critically important.

7. Geriatric Care Continuum

Geriatric clinical care involves multiple sites and levels of care. It differs from clinical care in other age groups as it often involves care not only in the ambulatory and inpatient settings, but also long term care and inpatient rehabilitation settings. In many developed countries, long term care of older adults includes nursing homes, assisted living facilities and continuing care retirement communities (CCRCs) which provide a range of services from ambulatory care for independent residents to assisted living and nursing home care, for those with significant cognitive and/or functional impairment. While these models of care are common, less than 5 percent of older adults in the United States live in nursing homes and about 2 percent in assisted living facilities [44]. These institutional long term care models are much less prevalent in African communities, with many older adults living in multi-generational family homes and majority of caregivers being family members. Several decades ago, in many African countries such as Nigeria, the few institutional nursing care homes that existed were mainly for older adults who were poor, with no family or for those with significant psychiatric issues [45]. With urbanization of many African communities and with many younger adults travelling to other countries for better economic opportunities, this trend is gradually changing. There are now more institutional care options for older African adults, particularly in larger cities. Home-based medical care is also gaining increasing popularity worldwide, with clinicians making house calls, particularly for frail older adults with significant mobility or cognitive issues. There may be some limitations in accessing this type of care in some African communities and developing countries, where poverty is prevalent and clinical resources are scarce [46].

8. Advance Care Planning

Advance care planning is a critical, yet often overlooked aspect of geriatric clinical care. It involves exploring patients' personal values, goals of medical care, including treatment modalities and end of life care, as well as appointing surrogate decision makers when there is loss of the ability to make health-related decisions. This process can be difficult for many patients and requires appropriate clinician communication with careful consideration of the patient's cultural beliefs, family relationships and social support network. With many adults of African ancestry, this can be especially difficult, depending on individual beliefs and preferences, which are often widely variable. So it is important for clinicians to carefully explore these beliefs and not rely on stereotypes. In some African cultures, discussions about end of life and death are considered bad omens and are simply not part of general discourse. While with some African American communities, mistrust of the medical system may influence goals of care decisions, sometimes leading to detrimental consequences to the patient. The various advance directive forms such as living will, durable power of attorney for health care (DPOA) and physician orders for life sustaining treatment (POLST) may also be confusing for some older adults and often times require careful explanation by the clinician. In some instances, it may be useful to have a close family member present. For some older African adults, it may be prudent to focus discussions on appointing a surrogate decision maker (DPOA) for future health-related situations, if decisions on end of life treatment and goals of medical care prove to be too difficult for the individual patient. It is very important for clinicians to explore these care preferences of older adults, preferably before they become sick or develop cognitive deficits.

References

[1] Joo JH, Jimenez DE, Xu J, Park M. Perspectives on Training Needs for Geriatric Mental Health Providers: Preparing to Serve a Diverse Older Adult Population. *Am J Geriatr Psychiatry.* 2019; 27(7):728-736.

[2] Noh H. Values important to terminally ill African American older adults in receiving hospice care. *J Soc Work End Life Palliat Care.* 2014; 10(4):338-55.

[3] Kataoka-Yahiro MR, McFarlane S, Koijane J, Li D. Culturally Competent Palliative and Hospice Care Training for Ethnically Diverse Staff in Long-Term Care Facilities. *Am J Hosp Palliat Care.* 2017; 34(4):335-346.

[4] Vaccaro JA, Huffman FG. Sex and Race/Ethnic Disparities in Food Security and Chronic Diseases in U.S. Older Adults *Gerontol Geriatr Med.* 2017; 30;3.

[5] Lindeman RD. Overview: renal physiology and pathophysiology of aging. *Am J Kidney Dis.* 1990; 16(4):275.

[6] King AC, Guralnik JM. Maximizing the potential of an aging population. *JAMA.* 2010; 304(17):1944-1945.

[7] Nelson ME, Rejeski WJ, Blair SN, Duncan PW, Judge JO, King AC et al. Physical activity and public health in older adults: recommendation from the American College of Sports Medicine and the American Heart Association. *Circulation.* 2007; 116(9):1094-1105.

[8] Maisto SA, Saitz R. Alcohol use disorders: screening and diagnosis. *Am J Addict.* 2003; 12 Suppl 1:S12.

[9] Kim EJ, Kim T, Conigliaro J, Liebschutz JM, Paasche-Orlow MK, Hanchate AD. Racial and Ethnic Disparities in Diagnosis of Chronic Medical Conditions in the USA. *J Gen Intern Med.* 2018; 33(7):1116-1123.

[10] Dooling KL, Guo A, Patel M, Lee GM, Moore K, Belongia EA et al. Recommendations of the Advisory Committee on Immunization Practices for Use of Herpes Zoster Vaccines. *MMWR Morb Mortal Wkly Rep*. 2018; 67(3):103-108.

[11] Nelson HD, Fu R, Cantor A, Pappas M, Daeges M, Humphrey L. Effectiveness of Breast Cancer Screening: Systematic Review and Meta-analysis to Update the 2009 U.S. Preventive Services Task Force Recommendation. *Ann Intern Med.* 2016; 164(4):244-255.

[12] Qaseem A, Barry MJ, Denberg TD, Owens DK, Shekelle P; Clinical Guidelines Committee of the American College of Physicians. Screening for prostate cancer: a guidance statement from the Clinical Guidelines Committee of the American College of Physicians. *Ann Intern Med.* 2013; 158(10):761-769.

[13] National Lung Screening Trial Research Team, Aberle DR, Adams AM, et al. Reduced lung-cancer mortality with low-dose computed tomographic screening. *N Engl J Med.* 2011; 365(5):395-409.

[14] Stevens GA, White RA, Flaxman SR, Price H, Jonas JB, Keeffe J et al. Vision Loss Expert Group. Global prevalence of vision impairment and blindness: magnitude and temporal trends, 1990-2010. *Ophthalmology.* 2013; 120(12):2377-2384.

[15] Moreland B, Kakara R, Henry A. Trends in Nonfatal Falls and Fall-Related Injuries Among Adults Aged ≥65 Years - United States, 2012-2018. *MMWR Morb Mortal Wkly Rep.* 2020; 10:69(27):875-881.

[16] Sattin RW, Lambert Huber DA, DeVito CA, Rodriguez JG, Ros A, Bacchelli S, Stevens JA, Waxweiler RJ. The incidence of fall injury events among the elderly in a defined population. *Am J Epidemiol.* 1990; 131(6):1028-37.

[17] Tinetti ME, Speechley M, Ginter SF. Risk factors for falls among elderly persons living in the community. *N Engl J Med.* 1988; 29:319(26):1701-7.

[18] Schoene D, Wu SM, Mikolaizak AS, Menant JC, Smith ST, Delbaere K, Lord SR. Discriminative ability and predictive validity of the timed up and go test in identifying older people who fall: systematic review and meta-analysis. *J Am Geriatr Soc.* 2013; 61(2):202-8.

[19] Tinetti, ME. Performance-Oriented Assessment of Mobility Problems in Elderly Patients. *J Am Geriatr Soc.* 1986; 34: 119-126.

[20] Deurenberg P, Yap M, van Staveren WA. Body mass index and percent body fat: a meta-analysis among different ethnic groups. *Int J Obes Relat Metab Disord.* 1998 Dec; 22(12):1164-71.

[21] Compston J, Cooper A, Cooper C, et al. UK clinical guideline for the prevention and treatment of osteoporosis. *Arch Osteoporos.* 2017; 12(1):43.

[22] Wallace JI, Schwartz RS, LaCroix AZ, Uhlmann RF, Pearlman RA. Involuntary weight loss in older outpatients: incidence and clinical significance. *J Am Geriatr Soc.* 1995 Apr; 43(4):329-37.

[23] Houston DK, Tooze JA, Garcia K, Visser M, Rubin S, Harris TB, Newman AB, Kritchevsky SB; Health ABC Study. Protein Intake and Mobility Limitation in Community-Dwelling Older Adults: the Health ABC Study. *J Am Geriatr Soc.* 2017 Aug; 65(8):1705-1711.

[24] Gil-Montoya JA, Ponce G, Sánchez Lara I, Barrios R, Llodra JC, Bravo M. Association of the oral health impact profile with malnutrition risk in Spanish elders. *Arch Gerontol Geriatr* 2013; 57:398–402.

[25] Naidoo I, Charlton KE, Esterhuizen TM, Cassim B. High risk of malnutrition associated with depressive symptoms in older South Africans living in KwaZulu-Natal, South Africa: a cross-sectional survey. *J Health Popul Nutr.* 2015; 33:19.

[26] Zawada ET Jr. Malnutrition in the elderly. Is it simply a matter of not eating enough? *Postgrad Med.* 1996 Jul; 100(1):207-8, 211-4, 220-2.

[27] Milne AC, Avenell A, Potter J. Meta-analysis: protein and energy supplementation in older people. *Ann Intern Med.* 2006 Jan 3; 144(1):37-48.

[28] Segers K, Surquin M. Can mirtazapine counteract the weight loss associated with Alzheimer disease? A retrospective open-label study. *Alzheimer Dis Assoc Disord.* 2014 Jul-Sep; 28(3):291-3.

[29] Bodenner D, Spencer T, Riggs AT, Redman C, Strunk B, Hughes T. A retrospective study of the association between megestrol acetate administration and mortality among nursing home residents with clinically significant weight loss. *Am J Geriatr Pharmacother.* 2007 Jun; 5(2):137-46.

[30] White HK, Petrie CD, Landschulz W, MacLean D, Taylor A, Lyles K et al. Capromorelin Study Group. Effects of an oral growth hormone secretagogue in older adults. *J Clin Endocrinol Metab.* 2009 Apr; 94(4):1198-206.

[31] Wee CC, Huskey KW, Ngo LH, Fowler-Brown A, Leveille SG, Mittlemen MA et al. Obesity, race, and risk for death or functional decline among Medicare beneficiaries: a cohort study. *Ann Intern Med.* 2011 May 17;154(10):645-55.

[32] Sims J, Browning C, Lundgren-Lindquist B, Kendig H. Urinary incontinence in a community sample of older adults: prevalence and impact on quality of life. *Disabil Rehabil.* 2011; 33(15-16):1389-98.

[33] Thom D. Variation in estimates of urinary incontinence prevalence in the community: effects of differences in definition, population characteristics, and study type. *J Am Geriatr Soc.* 1998 Apr;46(4):473-80.

[34] Schubert M, Schürch R, Boettger S, Garcia Nuñez D, Schwarz U, Bettex D et al. A hospital-wide evaluation of delirium prevalence and outcomes in acute care patients - a cohort study. *BMC Health Serv Res.* 2018 Jul 13; 18(1):550.

[35] Fiest KM, Roberts JI, Maxwell CJ, Hogan DB, Smith EE, Frolkis A et al. The Prevalence and Incidence of Dementia Due to Alzheimer's Disease: a Systematic Review and Meta-Analysis. *Can J Neurol Sci.* 2016 Apr; 43 Suppl 1:S51-82.

[36] World Health Organization (WHO). WHO scientific group on the assessment of osteoporosis at primary health care level: summary

meeting report. Available at: https://www.who.int/chp/topics/ Osteoporosis.pdf. Accessed October 26, 2020.

[37] Kaufman DW, Kelly JP, Rosenberg L, Anderson TE, Mitchell AA. Recent patterns of medication use in the ambulatory adult population of the United States: the Slone survey. *JAMA*. 2002 Jan 16; 287(3):337-44.

[38] Qato DM, Alexander GC, Conti RM, Johnson M, Schumm P, Lindau ST. Use of prescription and over-the-counter medications and dietary supplements among older adults in the United States. *JAMA*. 2008 Dec 24;300(24):2867-78.

[39] Budnitz DS, Lovegrove MC, Shehab N, Richards CL. Emergency hospitalizations for adverse drug events in older Americans. *N Engl J Med*. 2011 Nov 24;365(21):2002-12.

[40] van Heerden JA, Burger JR, Gerber JJ, Vlahović-Palčevski V. Prevalence of potentially serious drug-drug interactions among South African elderly private health sector patients using the Mimica Matanović/Vlahović-Palčevski protocol. *Int J Pharm Pract*. 2018 Apr; 26(2):156-164.

[41] By the 2019 American Geriatrics Society Beers Criteria® Update Expert Panel. American Geriatrics Society 2019 Updated AGS Beers Criteria® for Potentially Inappropriate Medication Use in Older Adults. *J Am Geriatr Soc*. 2019 Apr;67(4):674-694.

[42] Van Heerden JA, Burger JR, Gerber JJ. Inappropriate medicine prescribing in older South Africans: A cross-sectional analysis of medicine claims data. *S Afr Med J. 2016* Sep 9;106(10):1010-1016.

[43] Lutz BH, Miranda VIA, Bertoldi AD. Potentially inappropriate medications among older adults in Pelotas, Southern Brazil. *Rev Saude Publica*. 2017 Jun 22;51:52.

[44] Institute of Medicine (US) Food Forum. Providing Healthy and Safe Foods As We Age: Workshop Summary. Washington (DC): National Academies Press (US); 2010. 2, *Size and Demographics of Aging Populations*. Available from: https://www.ncbi.nlm.nih.gov/books/ NBK51841/ Accessed December 7, 2020.

[45] Akanji BO, Ogunniyi A, Baiyewu O. Healthcare or older persons, a country profile: Nigeria. *J Am Geriatr Soc* 2002; 50: 1289-1292.

[46] Balogun SA, Osi-Ogbu O. Geriatric House Calls: A Geriatrician- Led Clinical Experience in Sub-Saharan Africa. *Gerontology & Geriatric Research*. 2020 Epub: doi: 10.31487/j.GGR.2019.01.03.

In: Care of the Older African Adult
Editor: Seki A. Balogun
ISBN: 978-1-53619-295-7

Chapter 2

CARDIAC DISEASES IN OLDER AFRICAN ADULTS

Sula Mazimba[1,*] and Hunter Mwansa[2]
[1]Associate Professor of Medicine,
Division of Cardiovascular Medicine, University of Virginia,
Charlottesville, Virginia
[2]Clinical Instructor of Medicine
Department of Internal Medicine, OSF Saint Francis Medical Center,
University of Illinois College of Medicine, Peoria, Illinois

ABSTRACT

Cardiovascular disease (CVD) is the leading cause of death in Africa. Unlike in Western countries, CVD in Africa has a relatively earlier age of onset. The rise in traditional cardiovascular risk factors, such as hypertension and obesity, along with age related cardiovascular structural changes probably account for the shift in pattern and prevalence of CVD in older Africans. Rapid urbanization, adoption of unhealthy lifestyles such as diets rich in highly processed foods, physical inactivity, excessive alcohol consumption and tobacco use contribute to the clustering of CVD

* Corresponding Author's Email: SM8SD@hscmail.mcc.virginia.edu.

risk factors. Ischemic heart disease (IHD) attributable to these modifiable cardiovascular risks is rare but on the rise. Additionally, improved longevity related to widespread use of effective antiretroviral therapy (ART) modulates the interaction between traditional cardiovascular risks and HIV-related atherosclerosis, potentially amplifying IHD's contribution to the total CVD burden in Africa. Despite evidence of high CVD prevalence and poor outcomes in Africans, data on effective population-wide interventions is lacking. CVD in Africa poses unique healthcare delivery challenges due to lack of specialized care of cardiovascular diseases. There is therefore a pressing need to equip clinicians in Africa with knowledge and skills necessary to deliver quality care for patients with CVD.

Keywords: African, atherosclerosis, dilated cardiomyopathy, HIV-associated cardiomyopathy, non-ischemic cardiomyopathy, ischemic cardiomyopathy, ischemic heart disease, hypertension, stroke, heart failure, rheumatic heart disease, peripartum cardiomyopathy, atrial fibrillation, acute coronary syndromes

1. Epidemiology of CVD in Older Africans

Precise continental wide data on the incidence and prevalence of cardiovascular disease (CVD) in older Africans is sparse due to a general lack of robust CVD specific registries. In 2017, approximately 80% of the estimated 17.8 million global deaths attributable to CVD occurred in low- and middle-income countries; available data suggests a rapid rise of CVD prevalence and death in most African countries [1]. Conversely, CVD incidence as well as the attributable mortality have declined over the years in high-income countries [1]. CVD-related deaths almost doubled between 1990 and 2013, accounting for almost 1 million deaths (38.3% of non-communicable diseases and 11.3% of all causes of death) in Sub-Saharan Africa [2]. Rapid urbanization and the associated adoption of unhealthy lifestyles have led to an epidemiologic transition of non-communicable diseases in Africa. This is occurring even against a background of communicable diseases that have persisted in many regions of the continent. With the current epidemiologic transition, CVD prevalence in older Africans is projected to rise further. There is however regional heterogeneity in both pattern and distribution of CVD across Africa. Ischemic and hemorrhagic stroke, hypertensive heart disease (HHD), cardiomyopathy, and valvular heart disease (mainly rheumatic heart disease [RHD] and infective endocarditis [IE]) are the major contributors to cardiovascular morbidity and mortality in Africa. HHD- and stroke-related disability and death increase with advancing age, predominantly affecting patients aged 50 years and older.

2. Hypertension

2.1. Epidemiology

Hypertension is a leading cause of cardiovascular death and disability in Africa [3]. Hypertension contributes to greater than 50% of heart disease, stroke, and heart failure (HF). Low- and middle-income countries account for two-thirds of the global burden of hypertension, and Africa bears a disproportionate share of disease adjusted life years compared to other world regions [3]. Hypertension has a relatively earlier age of onset in Africans with peak incidence in middle age [4].

2.2. Definition and Risk Factors

Hypertension is defined as systolic blood pressure (SBP) ≥140 and/or diastolic blood pressure (DBP) ≥ 90 mmHg (Table 1) [5]. BP has a continuous relationship with cardiovascular events regardless of age and ethnicity [5]. However, SBP is a more potent and consistent predictor of cardiovascular outcomes after the age of 50 years [6]. Targeting lower blood pressure (BP) thresholds through pharmacologic and/or lifestyle interventions is associated with a reduction in CVD complications [5].

Table 1. Classification of hypertension

BP category	SBP (mmHg)	DBP (mmHg)
Normal	120-129	80-84
High normal	130-139	85-89
Grade 1 hypertension	140-159	90-99
Grade 2 hypertension	160-179	100-109
Grade 3 hypertension	≥ 180	≥ 110

BP: blood pressure; SBP: systolic blood pressure; DBP: diastolic blood pressure

Proper BP-measuring techniques using validated and well-calibrated BP-measuring devices is essential for the accurate diagnosis of hypertension. Home BP measurement (HBPM) in patients empowered with proper BP taking techniques and validated BP measuring devices can help confirm presence of white-coat hypertension (office BP > home BP by ≥ 20/10 mmHg) to avert unnecessary antihypertensive therapy. Ambulatory BP measurement (ABPM) is more reliable than HBPM but is not readily available in Africa. Both HBPM and ABPM are useful in patients suspected of white-coat hypertension, masked hypertension (normal office BP but elevated home or ambulatory BP), masked uncontrolled hypertension (controlled office BP but uncontrolled home or ambulatory BP), suspected medication-related hypotension, and resistant hypertension.

Hypertension often clusters with other cardiovascular risk factors such as advancing age, dyslipidemia, overweight (body mass index [BMI] 25 to 29.9), obesity [BMI ≥ 30], and diabetes which in aggregate augment risk for cardiovascular complications [4]. Epidemiologic studies of patients with hypertension in Africa have reported variable associations between hypertension and other established cardiovascular risk factors such as physical inactivity, excessive alcohol use, and nicotine use. The size and number of these studies limit generalizability. Co-existence of hypertension and other cardiovascular risk factors elevates the risk for death, stroke, and myocardial infarction [7]. Modification of these cardiovascular risks through pharmacologic and lifestyle measures attenuate CVD risk and death.

2.3. Clinical Management of Hypertension

2.3.1. Clinical Evaluation

The use of well-equilibrated blood pressure instruments is crucial for the proper diagnosis and management of hypertension. Documentation of elevated BP measurement, on a separate clinic visit, at least 1 week apart is essential for confirmation of hypertension in most patients. Identification of other CVD risk factors may enable clinicians to engage patients on behavioral modification strategies that may also aid in the control of hypertension. It is important to elicit on history, potential etiologies and contributors to the progression of hypertension. Identification of modifiable risks can help tailor therapeutic choices. A subset of older patients can benefit from further work up for secondary causes of hypertension. Older patients with a history of early onset (< 40 years) of grade 2-3 hypertension and sudden onset hypertension refractory to antihypertensive therapy should be evaluated for secondary hypertension. Clinical evaluation should identify potential etiologies of the hypertension and hypertension-mediated organ (kidney, heart, brain, eyes) damage.

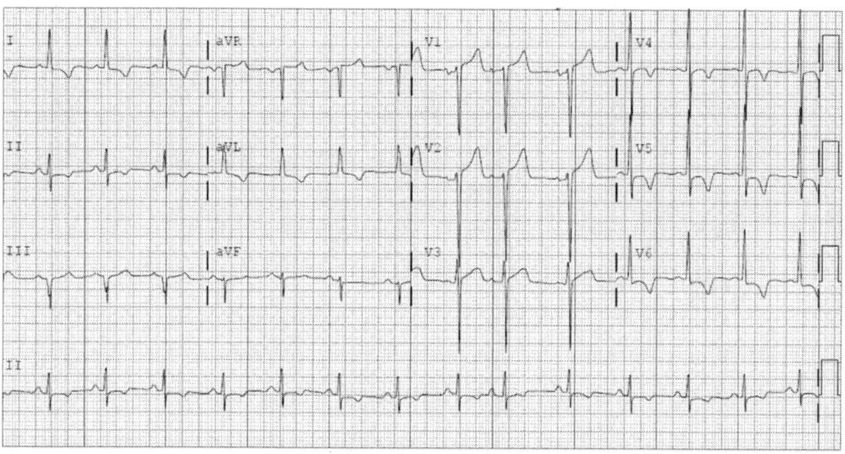

Figure 1. Electrocardiogram showing left ventricular hypertrophy.

Physical examination may reveal the presence of risks factors, potential causes of secondary hypertension, and hypertension-mediated organ damage

(HMOD). Initial evaluation should, whenever feasible, include an electrocardiogram (ECG) to exclude left ventricular hypertrophy (LVH, Figure 1) and arrhythmias, echocardiogram to assess cardiac structure and function if indicated (e.g., suspected HF), creatinine and glomerular filtration rate (GFR), urine microalbuminuria and fundoscopy.

2.3.2. Initiation of Antihypertensive Therapy

The World Health Organization/International Society of Hypertension (WHO/ISH) cardiovascular risk-prediction charts, which are based on age, sex, SBP, type 2 diabetes mellitus (T2DM) and total serum cholesterol, enable a reasonable quantification of cardiovascular risk and are applicable to patients with hypertension in Africa [8]. These charts are particularly useful in stratifying low-risk patients in order to determine appropriate therapeutic strategies as well as guide shared decision-making between clinicians and patients. The WHO/ISH risk-prediction charts were developed for WHO epidemiological sub-regions and not necessarily individual countries and in this sense, might limit their predictive accuracy in smaller African countries. Additionally, underestimation of total cardiovascular risk may occur in higher risk patients such as those with BP ≥ 160/110 mm Hg, total serum cholesterol ≥ 8 mmol/L (> 309 mg/dl), established CVD, and/or diabetic renal disease. In this regard, high-risk older adults with a 10-year-risk of heart attack or stroke ≥ 40% and established CVD (e.g., coronary artery disease, peripheral artery disease, cerebrovascular disease or transient ischemic attack, coronary or arterial revascularization, aortic aneurysm, aortic plaque with > 50% stenosis on imaging), diabetes with target organ damage, or severe chronic kidney disease (CKD) should preferably be managed using a combination of lifestyle measures and pharmacologic interventions. According to WHO/ISH guidelines, hypertensive patients with an estimated 10-year-risk of heart attack or stroke of 10% to < 20% may initially be managed with lifestyle measures. These recommendations were developed with a view to promoting cost-effective and efficient use of resources in resource-limited countries and can therefore be adapted to allow for more intensive therapy where feasible. High-risk older patients may benefit from initiation of BP lowering therapy to target goal BP < 140/90 mm Hg [9]. There is potential for harm if an aggressive BP treatment threshold (SBP < 120 mm Hg) is adopted in older high-risk patients with multiple comorbidities [10]. There is no consensus on actual BP targets for older patients, but clinicians should aim for stringent BP control (SBP 130-140 mmHg) while paying attention to a patient's clinical condition, frailty, and resource constraints.

2.3.3. Therapy

BP management involves the implementation of non-pharmacologic and pharmacologic strategies. Heterogeneity in clinical manifestations, susceptibility to hypertension-mediated end-organ injury, and clinical response to antihypertensive therapy exists within racial and ethnic subgroups. Africans are usually salt-sensitive and suffer hypertension characterized by low plasma renin levels and an attenuated response to renin-angiotensin-aldosterone system (RAAS) inhibition [11]. Reduced sodium intake (< 2g/day) is therefore associated with greater BP reductions in Africans than other racial/ethnic groups. Other lifestyle measures proven to lower BP include the Dietary Approaches to Stop Hypertension (DASH; diet rich in vegetables, fruits, whole grains and low-fat dairy products), weight loss, cessation of nicotine use, exercise, high potassium intake and reduced alcohol intake. Because of high salt-sensitivity and a blunted RAAS, Africans also achieve better BP reduction with thiazides, thiazide-like diuretics, and calcium channel blockers (CCB) and have the least BP response to RAAS-blocker monotherapy including beta-blockers (BB). The blunted BP response is however offset when RAAS-blockers are used in combination with other antihypertensive drug classes. A recent study found that amlodipine combined with either hydrochlorothiazide (HCTZ) or perindopril demonstrated better BP control than a combination of HCTZ and perindopril in a cohort of patients from sub-Saharan Africa (SSA) [12]. High-risk patients, particularly those with SBP>160 mmHg, often require combination therapy to achieve optimal BP control. Combination therapy using single-pill combinations (SPC) or polypills (fixed-dose combination of ≥1 antihypertensive agent, statin, and low-dose aspirin) decreases pill burden, improves medication adherence and BP control, and is associated with fewer adverse effects. Monotherapy alongside lifestyle measures is a reasonable option in low-risk and frail elderly patients. It is recommended that when making drug selection for the treatment of hypertension, consideration must be given to specific drug classes when certain co-existing medical conditions are present (e.g., CKD, HF, IHD). Angiotensin converting enzyme inhibitors (ACEI) and angiotensin receptor blockers (ARB) reduce proteinuria and slow CKD progression in patients with diabetic nephropathy. Beta-blockers (BB) have less effective BP-lowering effects than other antihypertensives but can help relieve angina and reduce coronary events. Patients with prior myocardial infarction (MI) and those with HF with reduced ejection fraction (LVEF < 40%) can initially be managed with RAAS-blockers, evidence-based beta-blockers (carvedilol, metoprolol succinate, bisoprolol) and aldosterone antagonists (AA) given their proven benefits in reducing mortality and hospitalization rates. Resistant hypertension (uncontrolled BP despite optimal doses of 3 different antihypertensive drug classes including a diuretic) may respond to the addition of low-dose spironolactone (amiloride or eplerenone, if intolerant to spironolactone), bisoprolol, or doxazosin [13]. One of the consequences of hypertension is the dreaded hypertensive crises characterized by BP ≥ 180/120 mmHg. Hypertensive urgency represents a crisis without hypertension-mediated organ damage (HMOD) and can be managed by either reinstituting oral antihypertensives where adherence is an issue or escalating antihypertensive dosages in patients with suboptimal BP control despite good adherence. Addressing causes of poor adherence to therapy and reinforcing lifestyle measures can also help better BP control. Hypertensive emergencies are characterized by HMOD and are associated with high mortality requiring prompt BP control to mitigate death and further HMOD. Examples of hypertensive emergencies include cerebrovascular accidents (ischemic or hemorrhagic strokes), encephalopathy, acute kidney injury (AKI), acute coronary syndromes (ACS), acute aortic syndromes (AAS), and acute HF. Because of cerebral autoregulation, BP should be lowered by no more than 20-25% in the first hour then to 160/110 mmHg in the next 2-6 hours following which oral antihypertensives can be reintroduced slowly to allow for a smooth transition off parenteral agents. ACS, pulmonary edema/acute HF, and AAS require immediate reduction of BP to < 140 mm Hg. Patients presenting with acute stroke are managed differently and require input from neurologists especially when systemic thrombolysis is an option. Available parenteral antihypertensive agents in Africa include labetalol, sodium nitroprusside, nitroglycerin, and hydralazine. Hydralazine has unpredictable BP-lowering effects making labetalol a more appropriate choice for most patients. A combination of labetalol and sodium nitroprusside is ideal for management of AAS while nitroglycerin or labetalol can be utilized in patients with ACS. Nitroglycerin or sodium nitroprusside in combination with loop diuretics can be used in patients with acute pulmonary edema.

3. Heart Failure

Heart failure (HF) is the final common pathway resulting from various injuries to cardiac tissues. The syndrome is characterized by a constellation of hypoperfusion and congestive symptoms due to structural and/or functional impairment of ventricular filling or ejection. Three major categories of HF are recognized namely, HF with reduced ejection fraction (HFrEF; EF $\leq$ 40%), mid-range ejection fraction (HFmrEF; EF 41-49), and preserved ejection fraction (HFpEF; EF $\geq$ 50%). Recent data suggests a rise in HFpEF and an equally poor prognosis among Africans [14]. Two of the most widely recognized HF classification systems are the New York Heart Association (NYHA) functional classification and American College of Cardiology/American Heart Association (ACC/AHA) staging system. The NYHA comprises classes I, II, III and IV, representing lack of HF symptoms with ordinary activity, HF symptoms with ordinary activity, HF symptoms with less than ordinary activity, and dyspnea at rest, respectively. The ACC/AHA staging recognizes the progressive nature of HF and constitutes stages A, B, C, and D. Stages A and B comprise asymptomatic patients with established HF risk factors (e.g., hypertension, diabetes) but no structural heart disease and asymptomatic patients with both risk factors and structural heart disease (e.g., left ventricular dysfunction, left ventricular hypertrophy, valvular disease), respectively. Stages C and D comprise stage B patients with current or prior HF symptoms and patients with refractory HF symptoms despite optimal guideline-directed medical therapy (GDMT), respectively.

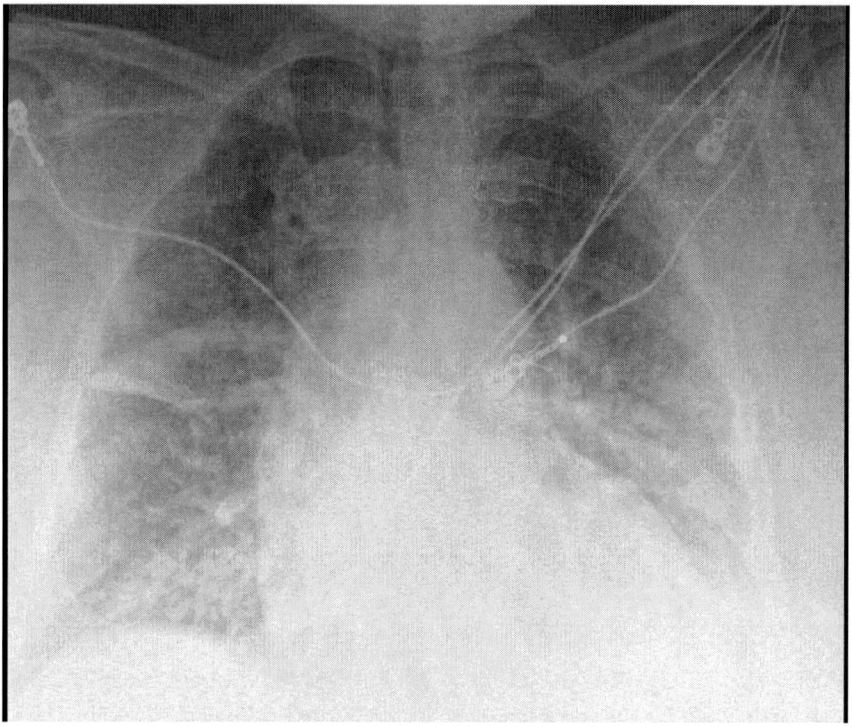

Antero-posterior chest x-ray of patient with heart failure reduced ejection fraction. Note the enlarged cardiac silhouette, bilateral pulmonary congestion and a small left pleural effusion.

Figure 2. Chest X-ray showing pulmonary edema.

3.1. Epidemiology

HF syndrome is a growing public health problem in Africa and incurs a huge health care burden. Non-ischemic causes including hypertension, cardiomyopathy and rheumatic heart disease (RHD) account for more than

75% of hospitalized HF in SSA [15]. Hypertension has emerged as the leading cause of HF, while ischemic heart disease (IHD) appears to be on the rise [15]. HF in Africa predominantly occurs in a relatively young patient population, with peak incidence in middle-age and about a decade earlier, compared to western countries where it predominantly affects persons aged 65 years and older

3.2. Clinical Presentation

HF has a highly variable clinical presentation. Generally, patients present with either new onset HF or decompensation of pre-existing chronic HF. Typical HF symptoms include effort intolerance, dyspnea, cough, orthopnea, paroxysmal nocturnal dyspnea, and/or edema. Diagnosis and management of HF may pose a huge challenge in developing countries, due to limited access to ancillary services, specifically, biomarkers and echocardiography. As such, HF diagnosis requires a high index of suspicion in patients presenting with suggestive symptoms. In patients with chronic HF, history should focus on possible causes of HF exacerbation such as poor adherence to medical therapy including sodium restriction, uncontrolled hypertension, concurrent pulmonary infections, and myocardial infarction. A physical examination focused on detection of congestive signs such as jugular venous distension (JVD), S3 gallop, hepatojugular reflux, tender hepatomegaly, ascites, pulmonary rales, and extremity edema is paramount. An ECG might reveal arrhythmias, conduction abnormalities, and cardiac ischemia. Chest x-ray may show cardiomegaly, pulmonary vascular congestion (Figure 2), and can at times help in identifying potential etiologies of HF. Patients with chronic HF may however have alveolar capillary wall thickening, pulmonary hypertension and well-developed lymphatic drainage leading to absence of pulmonary rales and radiographic vascular congestion. With limited access to brain natriuretic peptides and echocardiography, HF scores, tailored to identify congestive symptoms and signs of HF might prove particularly useful [16]. Whenever feasible, echocardiography should be performed to assess cardiac structure and function to help delineate HF categories and potential etiologies with varying implications for therapy. The NYHA functional classification can be a valuable clinical monitoring tool and should be used to gauge therapeutic response to HF therapies including diuretics.

3.3. Clinical Management of Stable HF

Broadly, the goals of therapy in HF are to improve quality of life and prolong survival. Unfortunately, HF occurs prematurely and presents in later stages of the disease (NYHA class IV) in most Africans [17]. Furthermore, suboptimal doses of guide-directed medical therapy (GDMT) is common in many regions of the continent. All patients with HFrEF must be on optimal doses of GDMT including a RAAS-blocker (ACEI or ARB when ACEI intolerant), beta-blocker, and aldosterone antagonist (AA) if indicated. ACEIs suppress the RAAS leading to vasodilatory and reverse remodeling effects on the cardiovascular system. ACEIs improve HF symptoms, readmission rates, and mortality [18]. ARBs block Angiotensin II receptors and have similar efficacy to ACEIs, and while scarce in Africa, should be utilized where ACEI intolerance exists. Beta-blockers have negative chronotropic effects that favorably attenuate cardiovascular effects of the maladaptive adrenergic overdrive characteristic of HF. Evidence-based beta-blockers (carvedilol, metoprolol succinate, bisoprolol) improve survival, event-free survival, readmission rates, and quality of life [19]. Aldosterone antagonists such as spironolactone improve mortality and HF readmissions even in older patients [20]. Ideally, HF patients should be on optimal doses of RAAS and beta-blockers before addition of an aldosterone antagonist. In addition, combination vasodilator therapy of hydralazine and isosorbide dinitrate improves morbidity and mortality in African patients with NYHA class III-IV HF and should be used in patients intolerant to RAAS-blockers and patients with refractory HF symptoms despite maximal tolerable doses of optimal GDMT (ACEI/ABR, beta-blocker, AA) [21]. Newer HF therapies such as angiotensin receptor blocker-neprilysin inhibitors and sodium-glucose cotransporter-2 inhibitors are not widely available in most parts of Africa due to high cost. When feasible, NYHA class II-III patients with chronic HF on optimal GDMT with left ventricular ejection fraction (LVEF) $\leq$ 35% must be referred to expert centers for Implantable Cardioverter-Defibrillator implantation to prevent sudden cardiac death. Some African countries have capabilities for cardiac resynchronization therapy (CRT), proven to reverse cardiac remodeling, improve HF morbidity, quality of life, and death. CRT is indicated in patients with symptomatic HFrEF (EF $\leq$ 35%, QRS interval $\geq$ 150ms, left bundle branch block, and sinus rhythm). Device-based management strategies in HF are hampered by cost, lack of infrastructure, and clinical expertise in these areas.

3.4. Management of Acute HF

Congestive symptoms are the main reason HF patients present acutely to seek care. Diuretics improve congestive symptoms and exercise tolerance but have no mortality benefit. The most widely used loop diuretic in many parts of Africa is furosemide. Given the prognostic value of congestion in HF, patients should achieve adequate diuresis before discharge. Improvement in exertional dyspnea, decrease in JVD, weight loss, and loss of initial paradoxical increase in BP with orthostasis constitute important clinical parameters for assessment of a patient's volume status before discharge [16]. Serum sodium and blood urea nitrogen (BUN) can also inform a patient's volume status with marked decreases and elevations, respectively, suggesting volume overload and poor outcomes. Normalization in sodium and BUN can generally be observed with good diuresis. Patients with cardiogenic shock (HF with clinical symptoms and signs of hypotension and global hypoperfusion such as encephalopathy, liver dysfunction, renal dysfunction, and cold extremities) may require inotropes/pressors such as norepinephrine, dopamine, and dobutamine. HF patients with cardiogenic shock are best managed in tertiary care centers with adequate infrastructure. Following adequate decongestion, hemodynamically stable patients should be started on GDMT at lower doses and up titrated as tolerated to target optimal doses reflected in clinical trials. Gradual optimization of beta-blockers over 1-2 weekly intervals may help avoid development of adherence limiting adverse effects. Age-related decline in renal function, complex drug pharmacokinetics including narrow therapeutic window and lack of access to drug monitoring predispose older Africans to digoxin toxicity. As such, Digoxin use may only be appropriate for symptomatic relief in select patients e.g., end-stage HF. Early follow-up and referrals for cardiac rehabilitation, whenever possible, may improve outcomes and functional status.

3.5. Specific Causes of HF in older Africans

3.5.1. Hypertensive Heart Disease

This relates to cardiac damage due to longstanding uncontrolled hypertension. Chronic uncontrolled hypertension leads to left ventricular hypertrophy (LVH) which can cause elevated end-diastolic pressure and diastolic dysfunction. Hypertensive HF is a diagnostic consideration in patients with documented HHD and HF symptoms. Besides reversal of LVH, antihypertensive therapy may improve HF morbidity and mortality. The overarching goals of therapy include optimal BP control and GDMT in patients with concurrent HFrEF.

3.5.2. Non-Ischemic Dilated Cardiomyopathy (DCM)

This is characterized by ventricular remodeling, dilatation, and compromised contractility in the absence of cardiovascular diseases such as hypertension and valvular heart disease. It is a heterogeneous group of heart muscle diseases with diverse etiologies and commonly causes HF [15] in SSA. An aggressive diagnostic strategy that includes coronary angiography and endomyocardial biopsy may reveal a cause of DCM in previously idiopathic cases. Arrhythmias, thromboembolism, and sudden cardiac death are common in DCM patients.

3.5.3. Familial Dilated Cardiomyopathy

Accounts for 25-50% of cardiomyopathies in general [22] but the prevalence in Africa is less clear. Gene mapping has revealed >40 disease genes and the predominant mode of transmission is autosomal dominant. These genes encode multiple cellular components and pathways which alter cardiomyocyte structure and function leading to apoptosis. Familial DCM has also been associated with HLA-DR1 and DRw10 in African subjects [23], findings that suggest a role of gene-mediated immune involvement. Exclusion of other causes of DCM in patients with a suggestive family history is key to identification of this disorder. While treated like other causes of HF, heart transplantation is a standard therapeutic option for patients with DCM and advanced HF (Figure. 3).

3.5.4. Peripartum Cardiomyopathy (PPCM)

Peripartum cardiomyopathy (PPCM) is a rare complication of pregnancy. It often presents as a dilated cardiomyopathy towards the end of pregnancy or within a few months postpartum [24]. Although this type of heart failure occurs in women of childbearing age, some patients do not recover, and it may persist as a cause of heart failure in older adults [25]. Left ventricular function recovery may occur in up to 42% of patients in some studies [26, 27]. Even so, there is evidence that the left ventricular contractile reserve remains poor and may be susceptible to increased loading conditions such as hypertension [28]. Withdrawal of guideline directed medical therapy is usually accompanied by higher rates of deterioration in the left ventricular function among those with previously recovered function [29]. The pathophysiologic mechanisms of PPCM are unclear but it has been suggested that an interplay of genetic, traditional cardiovascular risks, and vasculo-humoral factors drive its development. PPCM has a disproportionately higher prevalence in African women, particularly those with pre-eclampsia. Evidence of therapeutic benefit from prolactin inhibition [30] supports the possible role of hormones in the pathogenesis of the disease. Africans of color present with more severe disease (more depressed LVEF) and worse outcomes compared to other racial/ethnic groups. Older patients with residual/persistent left ventricular dysfunction following PPCM should be managed with evidence-based HF therapies including beta-blockers.

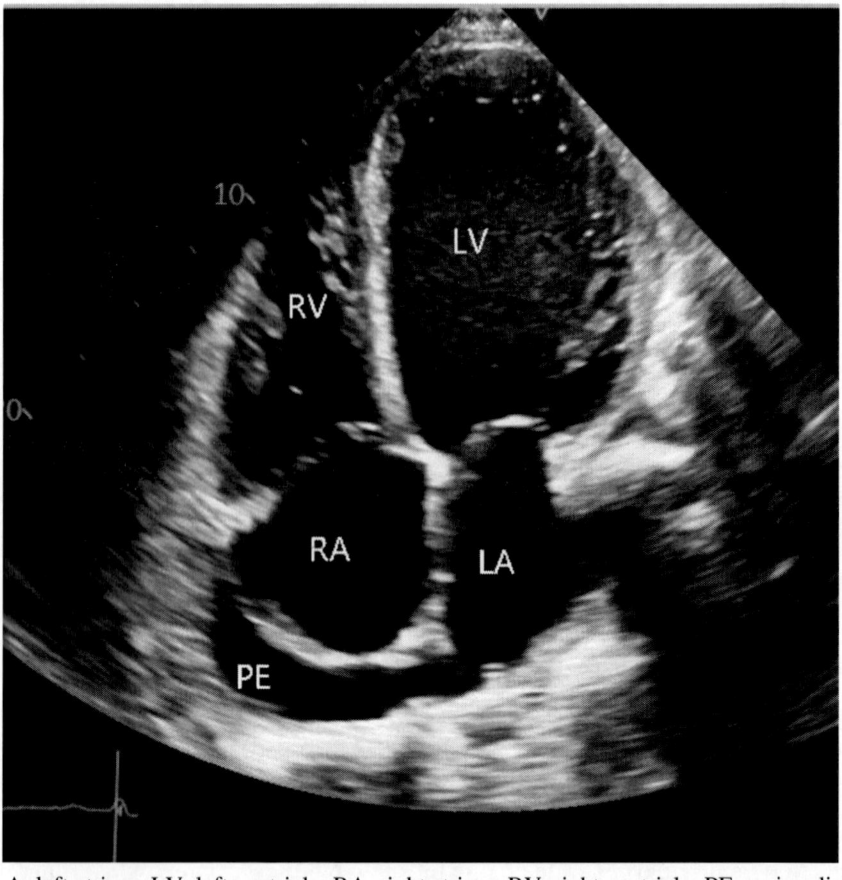

LA, left atrium; LV, left ventricle; RA, right atrium; RV, right ventricle; PE, pericardial effusion.

Figure 3. Apical-4 chamber view of familial dilated cardiomyopathy.

3.5.5. Alcoholic-Dilated Cardiomyopathy (ACM)

This is the most prevalent form of toxin-mediated cardiomyopathy, but studies on this HF syndrome are lacking in Africa. Alcohol causes dose-dependent cardiomyocyte damage and impairment of cardiac protein synthesis [31] in genetically susceptible individuals. Heavy and chronic alcoholics are at highest risk. Nonconventional traditional brews with varying alcohol concentrations and communal patterns of alcohol consumption make quantification of alcohol intake challenging in Africa. ACM can occur concurrently with nutritional cardiomyopathies such as thiamine deficiency mediated Wet Beriberi, but the two conditions are not related. Wet Beriberi is a form of high-output HF that responds to thiamine repletion. Alcohol contaminants may also play a role but their prevalence in traditional African brews has not been investigated. ACM is a diagnosis of exclusion and cessation of alcohol intake alongside other HF therapies can improve outcomes [31].

3.5.6. Rheumatic Heart Disease (RHD)

Ranks third among top causes of HF in Africa. It is a late sequelae of acute rheumatic fever (ARF), an inflammatory disease occurring 2-3 weeks following pharyngeal infection with group A β-hemolytic Streptococci in children. Carditis occurs in about 80% of individuals with ARF and 50% of affected patients subsequently develop chronic RHD. RHD commonly affects mitral and aortic valves; valvular regurgitation is the commonest manifestation in patients < 25 years whereas mitral stenosis and mixed valvular disease is more prevalent in older patients [32]. RHD leads to arrhythmias (commonly atrial fibrillation [AF]), infective endocarditis (IE), stroke, and symptomatic HF. The disease has a characteristically aggressive course and frequently causes premature death in Africa. RHD patients are usually asymptomatic until onset of LV dysfunction, pulmonary hypertension, and AF at which time HF symptoms dominate. Patients with severe mitral stenosis may also present with hemoptysis. Physical exam findings of mitral stenotic and/or regurgitant murmurs and aortic regurgitation in patients with a history of ARF suggest RHD but have low sensitivity. Echocardiography is more sensitive and specific than auscultation and may pick subclinical RHD (RHD without a clinically pathologic cardiac murmur, Figure 4) [33]. The therapeutic impact of identifying subclinical disease remains unclear. Echocardiographic assessments for RHD fall into three categories: 'definite RHD', 'borderline RHD', and 'normal' with the first two categories having four and three subcategories to reflect patterns of valvular involvement [33]. These guidelines were developed to enable early identification of RHD in individuals with no clear history of ARF who could potentially be enrolled in secondary prophylaxis programs to determine the role of echocardiographic screening in RHD control. RHD patients must receive 2-4 weekly intramuscular penicillin doses for secondary prevention of recurrent RF to prevent progression of RHD. Patients with concurrent HF and AF may benefit from adjunctive GDMT and anticoagulation with coumadin, respectively. Patients with infective endocarditis (IE) usually require a combination of parenteral antibiotic therapy and valve surgery. Surgical valve repair or replacement offers definitive therapy, but access is limited. Valvuloplasty might be a good option in poor surgical candidates.

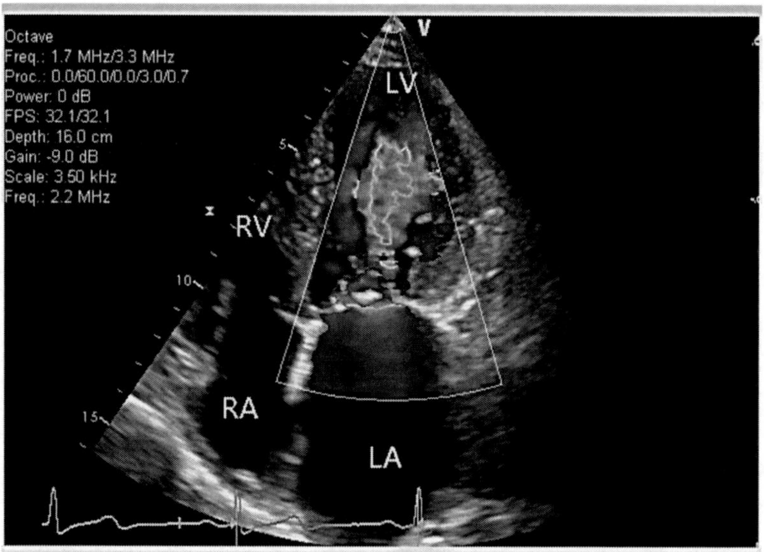

LA, left atrium; LV, left ventricle; RA, right atrium; RV, right ventricle

Figure 4. Apical-4 chamber view of severe rheumatic mitral stenosis.

3.5.7. Tuberculous (TB) Pericardial Diseases

Tuberculosis is the predominant cause of pericardial diseases in Africa [34]. Human Immunodeficiency Virus (HIV) co-infection is associated with worse outcomes including death. Patients with TB pericarditis and concomitant HIV have a mortality as high as 40% compared to 17% in HIV-seronegative patients [34]. In patients with mycobacterial infection, pericardial involvement can occur through hematogenous spread, retrograde spread via lymphatics, and/or contiguous spread from lungs and pleura. The intensity of the immune response to TB antigens within the pericardium parallels the morbidity seen in immunocompetent patients. TB pericarditis in HIV patients represents a more aggressive disease possibly influenced by the extent of immunosuppression due to HIV. Immunosuppression favors hematogenous dissemination of TB to the pericardium while immunocompetence favors spread via lymphatics. The spectrum of disease varies from effusive pericarditis (79.5%), effusive constrictive pericarditis (15.1%), and myopericarditis (13%). Interestingly, HIV co-infection is associated with a lower incidence of constrictive pericarditis [35]. Patients can present with pleurisy, fever, night sweats, anorexia, weight loss, and HF symptoms. Physical examination might reveal pericardial friction rub in early disease, distant heart sounds, pulsus paradoxus, JVD, hepatomegaly, and edema. ECG changes include diffuse ST-segment-elevation and PR-segment depression in patients with pericarditis and electrical alternans in those with significant pericardial effusions. An enlarged and globular cardiac silhouette on chest radiograph suggests pericardial effusion. Echocardiography can promptly identify cardiac tamponade and effusive and restrictive physiology (Figure 5).

Pericardiocentesis coupled with biochemistry, white cell counts, cytology, bacteria, and mycobacterial cultures can help determine the etiology of pericarditis. Where chemistry is not available, a serosanguinous exudate having elevated leukocytes with lymphocytic and monocytic pleocytosis is suggestive of TB pericarditis. Confirmation of infection is particularly challenging because microbiologic yield from pericardial fluid analysis and even targeted pericardial biopsy is generally low [36]. Adjunct tests are important to exclude other causes of exudative pericardial effusions such as malignancy.

Patients with tamponade require emergent pericardiocentesis. TB pericarditis is treated with combination anti-tuberculous chemotherapy. Corticosteroids decrease incidence of constrictive pericarditis but are associated with a 3-fold higher risk of HIV-associated cancer [37], and should therefore be avoided in HIV patients. Constrictive disease may require surgical decortication of the pericardium to relieve symptoms.

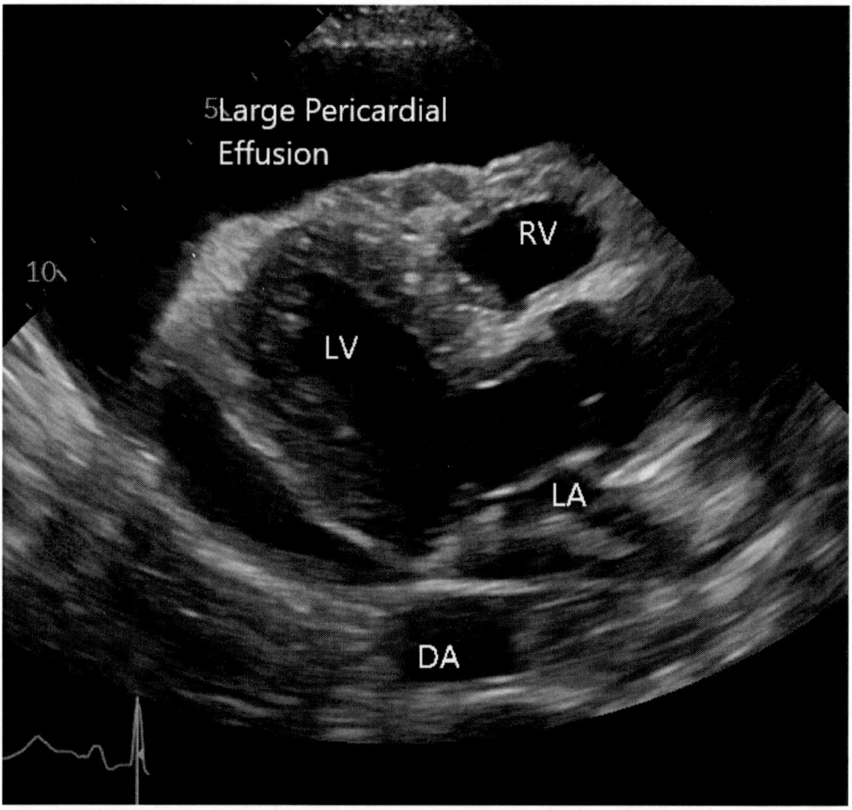

DA, descending aorta; LA, left atrium; LV left ventricle; RV, right ventricle

Figure 5. Parasternal view of large pericardial effusion.

3.5.8. Non-ischemic HIV-associated Cardiomyopathy

HIV-related myocardial damage causes both asymptomatic and symptomatic cardiac disease. Epidemiologically, the disease has evolved from a predominantly symptomatic DCM that characterized the pre-antiretroviral therapy era to a predominantly asymptomatic disease with variable cardiac manifestations including focal myocarditis, LV and right ventricular (RV) systolic and diastolic dysfunction [38]. Its prevalence is highly variable and appears to have a relation with access to antiretroviral therapy (ART). In the Heart of Soweto study, 38% of all HIV patients, of whom 54% were on ART, had HIV-associated cardiomyopathy and only 2.6% of HIV patients in the THESUS-HF study had HIV-associated cardiomyopathy as a cause of their HF [38], representing a decline in prevalence with more widespread use of ART [15]. Interpretation of these study findings requires caution because the Heart of Soweto registry findings may have limited generalizability and the THESUS-HF study was a multinational registry that enrolled hospitalized patients only. The etiology of non-ischemic HIV-associated cardiomyopathy is likely multifactorial and suggested mechanisms include an interplay of myocarditis and drug toxicity. First, despite a lack of CD4 cells on cardiomyocytes, cardiotropic viruses such as Epstein Barr Virus appear to promote HIV invasion of cardiomyocytes leading to myocarditis [38]. Second, HIV creates a proinflammatory milieu that causes myocardial inflammation and endothelial dysfunction even in patients on ART. Third, increased autoantibody production due to increased B-cell stimulation in HIV patients can cause myocarditis. Fourth, ART can cause direct myocardial injury (e.g., zidovudine) and cardiac steatosis (e.g., protease inhibitors).

In the ART era, HIV-associated cardiomyopathy is mostly asymptomatic and predominantly presents with diastolic dysfunction. DCM is usually found in symptomatic patients and portends poor outcomes [38]. HIV-associated cardiomyopathy is acquired immunodeficient syndrome (AIDS)-defining and as such affected patients require ART. ART may ameliorate cardiac dysfunction through restoration of immunity and viral suppression [38]. Selection of ART regimens with no proven or minimal cardiac adverse effects is key. And clinicians must watch for potential drug-drug interactions. Standard HF therapies in the absence of dedicated randomized clinical trials is reasonable when indicated.

3.5.9. Right Heart Failure

Right heart failure (RHF) is a major contributor to cases of the HF syndrome in Africa. Its prevalence in Africa is heterogeneous with disproportionately higher numbers than observed in high-income countries.

It can occur alone or in combination with left ventricular failure. In Africa, isolated RHF commonly follows pulmonary hypertension (defined as an elevated mean pulmonary artery pressure [mPAP] ≥25 mmHg at rest as measured by right heart catheterization [RHC]) that arises from chronic lung disease related to endemic pulmonary tuberculosis, restrictive lung disease, chronic obstructive pulmonary disease (COPD), chronic thromboembolic pulmonary hypertension (CTEPH), HIV, hemoglobinopathies (such as sickle cell disease), and schistosomiasis. It is unclear what role genetic and environmental factors (e.g., air pollutants) play in the etiology of pulmonary hypertension and RHF in Africa. Pulmonary hypertension is characterized by increased pulmonary vascular resistance and unfavorable right ventricular (RV) loading conditions which if sustained result in RV dilation and failure. Because of ventricular interdependence, RHF ultimately leads to LV dysfunction and failure. Isolated RHF predominantly presents with congestive symptoms. Clinical history may suggest the etiology of pulmonary hypertension and RHF. Characteristically, an accentuated S2 and diastolic and systolic murmurs of pulmonic and tricuspid regurgitation, respectively, may be present. Echocardiography helps screen for pulmonary hypertension and presence of left heart disease. Echocardiography may underestimate pulmonary artery systolic pressures but has a moderate sensitivity and specificity for pulmonary hypertension [39]. Further evaluation with chest x-ray, high resolution CT thorax, and pulmonary function tests including diffusion lung capacity for carbon monoxide can help unmask COPD and interstitial lung diseases (ILD). Management of patients with significant left heart disease but without severe pulmonary hypertension focuses on addressing the underlying left heart disease. COPD and ILD patients require therapies that address these lung conditions. A ventilation/perfusion (V/Q) scan can help exclude CTEPH in patients with no significant left heart and/or lung disease. RHC is not widely available in Africa but is the gold standard for diagnosis of pulmonary hypertension. Referral to tertiary care centers with CTEPH and severe pulmonary HTN and RHF expertise is beneficial whenever feasible. Judicious use of diuretics is advised to avoid compromising preload and cardiac output in patients with isolated RHF.

3.5.10. Ischemic Heart Disease

This is rarely a cause of HF in Africa. It accounted for HF in 7.7% of patients compared to 45.4% attributable to hypertension in the THESUS-HF study [15], representing an upward trajectory from 2% in 2005. This is likely an underestimate of the true burden of IHD at a population level because case detection might be limited by access to care. Adoption of unhealthy lifestyles such as unhealthy diets, nicotine use, excessive alcohol consumption, physical inactivity, and improved longevity partly account for the increase in IHD. The additional burden can be attributed to the high prevalence of HIV in Africa (70% of global burden) since HIV infection elevates risk for IHD. Multiple factors explain the heightened risk for IHD in patients with concomitant HIV: high prevalence of traditional cardiovascular risks in HIV patients; adverse ART effects (e.g., dyslipidemia and endothelial dysfunction); HIV-related inflammation and immune activation leading to a proatherogenic and procoagulant state; and chronic platelet activation leading to thrombosis [40].

Patients may present with either stable angina (dyspnea or exertional chest pain without ECG changes or elevation in cardiac enzymes) or acute coronary syndromes [ACS] (unstable angina, non-ST-segment-elevation myocardial infarction [NSTEMI] and ST-segment-elevation myocardial infarction [STEMI]). Unstable angina typically presents with chest pain at rest and/or dyspnea with or without ischemic ECG changes and non-elevated cardiac enzymes. NSTEMI presents similarly to unstable angina but is accompanied by elevated cardiac enzymes. STEMI classically presents with ST elevation $\geq$ 1 mm in 2 contiguous leads with or without elevated cardiac enzymes. Some patients may have coronary occlusion without classic ST-elevation (e.g., left bundle branch block, hyperacute T-waves, isolated ST-depression in anterior leads). STEMI diagnosis within 12 hours of symptom onset requires emergent reperfusion therapy. Generally, initial therapy requires administration of antiplatelet therapy (e.g., aspirin and clopidogrel), anticoagulation with heparin, statins, nitroglycerin, morphine, and/or beta-blocker therapy in absence of contraindications (HF, bradycardia, hypotension). Percutaneous coronary intervention (PCI) instituted within 120 minutes of STEMI diagnosis is superior in outcomes to medical thrombolysis. PCI is not widely available in Africa and, even when available, transfer to PCI-capable facilities may take > 120 minutes making fibrinolysis more pragmatic than PCI. Stable angina can be diagnosed with exercise stress testing. Beta-blockers, non-dihydropyridine calcium channel blockers, and long-acting nitrates help relieve angina symptoms. Concurrent ischemic cardiomyopathy and HFrEF require GDMT. Long-term management of IHD patients must also address cardiovascular risk reduction through adoption of health lifestyle interventions including weight loss through dietary measures and exercise, low salt intake, avoidance of nicotine use, and excessive alcohol consumption.

REFERENCES

[1] GBD 2017 Causes of Death Collaborators (2018) Global, regional, and national age-sex-specific mortality for 282 causes of death in 195 countries and territories, 1980-2017: a systematic analysis for the Global Burden of Disease Study 2017. *Lancet*, 392, 1736–1788.

[2] Mensah, GA; Roth, GA; Sampson, UK; Moran, AE; Feigin, VL; Forouzanfar, MH; et al. GBD 2013 Mortality and Causes of Death Collaborators. Mortality from cardiovascular diseases in sub-Saharan Africa; 1990-2013: a systematic analysis of data from the Global Burden of Disease Study 2013. *Cardiovasc J Afr.*, 2015 Mar-Apr, 26(2 Suppl 1), S6-10. doi: 10.5830/CVJA-2015-036. PMID: 25962950, PMCID: PMC4557490.

[3] *Institute for Health Metrics and Evaluation, 2015 University of Washington.* http://vizhub.healthdata.org/gbd-compare/. Accessed December 22, 2015.

[4] Bosu, WK; Aheto, JMK; Zucchelli, E; Reilly, ST. Determinants of systemic hypertension in older adults in Africa: a systematic review. *BMC Cardiovascular Disorders*, (2019), 19:173. https://doi.org/10.1186/s12872-019-1147-7

[5] Williams, B; Mancia, G; Spiering, W; et al. ESC Scientific Document Group, 2018 ESC/ESH Guidelines for the management of arterial

hypertension: The Task Force for the management of arterial hypertension of the European Society of Cardiology (ESC) and the European Society of Hypertension (ESH), *European Heart Journal*, Volume 39, Issue 33, 01 September 2018, Pages 3021–3104.

[6] Vishram, JK; Borglykke, A; Andreasen, AH; et al. MORGAM Project. Impact of age on the importance of systolic and diastolic blood pressures for stroke risk: the Monica, Risk, Genetics, Archiving, and Monograph (MORGAM) project. *Hypertension*, 2012, 60, 1117–1123.

[7] Egan, BM; Li, J; Hutchison, FN; et al. Hypertension in the United States, 1999 to 2012: progress toward Healthy People 2020 goals. *Circulation.*, 2014, 130, 1692-9.

[8] The WHO CVD Risk Chart Working Group. World Health Organization cardiovascular disease risk charts: revised models to estimate risk in 21 global regions. *Lancet Glob Health.*, 2019 Oct, 7(10), e1332–e1345.

[9] Brunstrom, M; Carlberg, B. Association of blood pressure lowering with mortality and cardiovascular disease across blood pressure levels: a systematic review and meta-analysis. *JAMA Intern Med*, 2018, 178, 28–36.

[10] Bohm, M; Schumacher, H; Teo, KK; et al. Achieved blood pressure and cardiovascular outcomes in high-risk patients: results from ONTARGET and TRANSCEND trials. *Lancet*, 2017, 389, 2226–2237.

[11] Brown, MJ. Hypertension and ethnic group. *BMJ.*, 2006, Apr 8, 332(7545), 833–836.

[12] Ojji, DB; Mayosi, B; Francis, V; et al., CREOLE Study Investigators. Comparison of dual therapies for lowering blood pressure in black Africans. *N Engl J Med.*, 2019, 380, 2429-39.

[13] Williams, B; MacDonald, TM; Morant, S; et al. British Hypertension Society's PATHWAY Studies Group. Spironolactone versus placebo, bisoprolol, and doxazosin to determine the optimal treatment for drug-resistant hypertension (PATHWAY-2): a randomised; double-blind, crossover trial. *Lancet*, 2015, 386, 2059–2068.

[14] Abebe, TB; Gebreyohannes, EA; Tefera, YG; Abegaz, TM. Patients with HFpEF and HFrEF have different clinical characteristics but similar prognosisa retrospective cohort study. *BMC Cardiovasc Disord*, 2016, 16, 232.

[15] Damasceno, A; Mayosi, BM; Sani, M; et al. The causes, treatment, and outcome of acute heart failure in 1006 Africans from 9 countries. *Arch Intern Med.*, 2012, 172, 1386–94.

[16] Gheorghiade, M; Follath, F; Ponikowski, P; et al. Assessing and grading congestion in acute heart failure: a scientific statement from the acute heart failure committee of the heart failure association of the European Society of Cardiology and endorsed by the European Society of Intensive Care Medicine. *Euro J Heart Fail.*, 2010 May, 12(5), 423-33.

[17] Dokainish, H; Teo, K; Zhu, J; et al. Heart failure in Africa, Asia, the Middle East and South America the INTER-CHF study. *Int J Cardiol*, 2016, 204, 133–41.

[18] Effect of enalapril on survival in patients with reduced left ventricular ejection fractions and congestive heart failure. The SOLVD Investigators. *N Engl J Med.*, 1991, 325, 293–302.

[19] Bristow, M. Beta-adrenergic receptor blockade in chronic heart failure. *Circulation*, 2000, 101, 558-569.

[20] Bayoumi, E; Lam, PH; Dooley, DJ; et al. Spironolactone and Outcomes in Older Patients with Heart Failure and Reduced Ejection Fraction. *Am J Med.*, 2019 January, 132(1), 71–80. e1. doi: 10.1016/ j.amjmed.2018.09.011.

[21] Taylor, AL; Ziesche, S; Yancy, C; et al. Combination of isosorbide dinitrate and hydralazine in blacks with heart failure. *N Engl J Med.*, 2004, 351, 2049-57.

[22] Watkins, H; Ashrafian, H; Redwood, C. Inherited cardiomyopathies. *N Engl J Med.*, 2011 Apr 28, 364(17), 1643-56.

[23] Khogali, SS; Mayosi, BM; Beattie, JM; et al. A common mitochondrial DNA variant associated with susceptibility to dilated cardiomyopathy in two different populations. *Lancet.*, 2001 Apr 21, 357(9264), 1265-7.

[24] Sliwa, K; Hilfiker-Kleiner, D; Petrie, MC; et al., Heart Failure Association of the European Society of Cardiology Working Group on Peripartum Cardiomyopathy. Current state of knowledge on etiology, diagnosis, management, and therapy of peripartum cardiomyopathy: a position statement from the Heart Failure Association of the European Society of Cardiology Working Group on peripartum cardiomyopathy. *Eur J Heart Fail*., 2010, 12, 767-78.

[25] Karaye, KM; Sa'idu, H; Balarabe, SA; et al. Clinical Features and Outcomes of Peripartum Cardiomyopathy in Nigeria. *J Am Coll Cardiol*, 2020, 76, 2352-2364.

[26] Pillarisetti, J; Kondur, A; Alani, A; et al. Peripartum Cardiomyopathy: Predictors of Recovery and Current State of Implantable Cardioverter-Defibrillator Use. *J Am Coll Cardiol*., 2014 Jul, 63 (25-Part-A), 2831–2839.

[27] Blauwet, LA; Libhaber, E; Forster, O; et al. Predictors of outcome in 176 South African patients with peripartum cardiomyopathy. *Heart*, 2013, 99, 308-313.

[28] Lampert, MB; Lynn, W; Hibbard, J; et al. Contractile reserve in patients with peripartum cardiomyopathy and recovered left ventricular function. *American Journal of Obstetrics and Gynecology*, Volume 176, Issue 1, Part 1, January 1997, Pages 189-195.

[29] Halliday, BP; Wassall, R; Lota, AS; et al. Withdrawal of pharmacological treatment for heart failure in patients with recovered dilated cardiomyopathy (TRED-HF): an open-label, pilot, randomised trial. *Lancet*, 2018, 393, 61–73.

[30] Haghikia, A; Podewski, E; Libhaber, E; et al. Phenotyping and outcome on contemporary management in a German cohort of patients with peripartum cardiomyopathy. *Basic Res Cardiol*., 2013, 108, 366.

[31] Joaquim Fernández-Solà. *The Effects of Ethanol on the Heart: Alcoholic Cardiomyopathy*. 2020 Feb 22, 12(2), 572.

[32] Sliwa, K; Carrington, M; Mayosi, BM; Zigiriadis, E; Mvungi, R; Stewart, S. Incidence and characteristics of newly diagnosed rheumatic heart disease in urban African adults: insights from the heart of Soweto study. *Eur Heart J*., 2010 Mar, 31(6), 719-27.

[33] Reményi, B; Wilson, N; Steer, A; et al. World Heart Federation criteria for echocardiographic diagnosis of rheumatic heart disease—an evidence-based guideline. *Nat Rev Cardiol.*, 2012 Feb 28, 9(5), 297-309.

[34] Ntsekhe, M; Mayosi, BM. Tuberculous pericarditis with and without HIV. *Heart Fail.*, 2013, Rev 18, 367–373.

[35] Ntsekhe, M; Wiysonge, CS; Gumedze, F; Maartens, G; Commerford, PJ; Volmink, JA; et al. (2008) HIV Infection Is Associated with a Lower Incidence of Constriction in Presumed Tuberculous Pericarditis: A Prospective Observational Study. *PLoS ONE*, 3(6), e2253. https://doi.org/10.1371/journal.pone.0002253.

[36] Sagristà-Sauleda, J; Mercé, AS; Soler-Soler, J. Diagnosis and management of pericardial effusion. *World J Cardiol.*, 2011, 3(5), 135–143.

[37] Mayosi, BM; Ntsekhe, M; Bosch, J; et al. and for the IMPI Trial Investigators. Prednisolone and Mycobacterium indicus pranii in tuberculous pericarditis. *N Engl J Med*, 371, (2014), pp. 1121-1130.

[38] Manga, P; McCutcheon, K; Tsabedze, N; Vachiat, A; Zachariah, D. HIV and Nonischemic Heart Disease. *J Am Coll Cardiol.*, 2017 Jan, 69 (1), 83-91.

[39] Janda, S; Shahidi, N; Gin, K; Swiston, J. Diagnostic accuracy of echocardiography for pulmonary hypertension: a systematic review and meta-analysis. *Heart.*, 2011 Apr, 97(8), 612-22.

[40] Vachiat, A; McCutcheon, K; Tsabedze, N; Zachariah, D; Manga, P. HIV and Ischemic Heart Disease. *J Am Coll Cardiol.*, 2017 Jan, 69 (1) 73-82.

In: Care of the Older African Adult
Editor: Seki A. Balogun
ISBN: 978-1-53619-295-7

Chapter 3

KIDNEY DISEASES IN OLDER AFRICAN ADULTS

Emaad M Abdel Rahman[1,*], Faruk Turgut[2,†] and Seki A. Balogun[3,‡]

[1]Professor, Internal Medicine, Division of Nephrology, University of Virginia Health System, Charlottesville, VA, US
[2]Professor, Internal Medicine, Division of Nephrology, Tayfur Ata Sokmen Faculty of Medicine, Hatay Mustafa Kemal University, Serinyol, Antakya, Hatay, Turkey
[3]Associate Professor, Internal Medicine, Division of General Medicine, Geriatrics and Palliative Care, University of Virginia Health System, Charlottesville, VA, US

ABSTRACT

Kidney diseases are common in older African adults. With aging, the kidneys are among the most significantly affected organs in the human

* Corresponding Author's Email: ea6n@virginia.edu.
† Corresponding Author's Email: turgutfaruk@yahoo.com.
‡ Corresponding Author's Email: sab2s@virginia.edu.

body, with both structural and functional changes that make them more susceptible to any additional injury. Many older African adults develop chronic kidney disease (CKD) from medical conditions such as hypertension, diabetes mellitus similar to populations in other parts of the world. However, the higher incidence of primary and infection induced glomerular diseases leading to kidney injury, make kidney diseases very prevalent in the older African population. Endemic infections such as human immunodeficiency virus (HIV), diarrheal diseases, malaria and the common use of herbal or traditional medicines which are often nephrotoxic, lead to acute kidney injury (AKI) and confer unique characteristics that define kidney diseases in older African adults. High poverty rates and inadequate access to optimal medical care in most of Africa also greatly contribute to development of kidney diseases, particularly CKD. Knowledge of the unique characteristics of these patients with its accompanying challenges is of paramount importance in providing optimal medical care for this vulnerable subset of the population. In this chapter, we review the different patterns and management of kidney diseases in older African adults, as well as outlining normal age-related anatomical and physiologic changes in kidney function.

Keywords: acute kidney injury, chronic kidney disease, glomerular filtration rate, nephrotoxins, hematuria, nephrosclerosis, urinary tract infection, hemodialysis, peritoneal dialysis, renal transplant

1. Epidemiology of Older Adults and Kidney Diseases in Africa

Kidney diseases are prevalent in Africa. With an average life expectancy of 61 years in males and 64 years in females across the continent [1], the majority of kidney diseases occur in 20-50 year olds. Many develop chronic kidney disease (CKD) primarily from hypertension, primary and infection induced glomerular diseases, and diabetes mellitus [2]. There is limited statistical data on the prevalence of kidney diseases in Africa, though it is estimated that 200-300 persons per million of the general African population have CKD [3].With the growing number of aging population in Africa along with the increasing prevalence of chronic conditions such as hypertension and diabetes mellitus, it is expected that the prevalence of the renal diseases in Africa will continue to rise. High poverty rates and lack of access to optimal medical care in most of Africa also greatly contribute to development of kidney diseases, particularly CKD [4].

2. Characteristics of Kidney Diseases in Africa

While kidney diseases in Africa mirror kidney diseases in many places in the world, there are some unique characteristics that define kidney diseases in the continent.

Pattern of acute kidney injury (AKI) disease in Africa takes a different shape than in the developed countries. The high prevalence of certain diseases like human immunodeficiency virus [HIV]-related AKI in sub-Saharan Africa, diarrheal diseases, malaria, surgical complications and presence of nephrotoxins offers a unique presentation of AKI in this continent. Other factors also contribute to the uniqueness of AKI presentation in Africa such as the late presentation of patients to health care facilities, and the lack of resources to support patients with established AKI [5].

In addition, the large consumption of herbal or traditional medicines in Africa without governmental regulation or pharmacological supervision in many African countries contributes to nephrotoxicity and AKI. Drug-drug interactions may also contribute to nephrotoxicity and AKI. Adibe et al. [6] retrospectively studied CKD patients in South East Nigeria and noted 749 cases of drug-drug interactions among 169 patients resulting in nephrotoxicity and AKI. The most common drug-drug interaction being lasix and lisinopril.

Unfortunately, reliable statistics about the incidence of AKI are lacking in many African countries. Some available data show the incidence of AKI in hospitalized patients in Africa ranging from 0.3 to 1.9% in adults, with 70 and 90% of cases of AKI being community acquired. The mortality associated with AKI in adults in Africa ranges from 11.5 to 43.5%, with a different pattern compared to the AKI-associated mortality in developed countries. In Africa, unlike in developed countries, the use of antiretroviral therapy (ART) in HIV-1-infected AKI patients is associated with a 6-fold higher risk of in-hospital mortality [7].

Similarly, hematuria in Africa presents with unique features. Pereira et al. [8] noted that the presence of intermittent terminal hematuria in African patients should lead to the suspicion of vesical schistosomiasis as the first diagnostic option. Another cause of hematuria in sub-Saharan Africa, is sickle cell disease (SCD) [9]. Clinically significant renal involvement which tends to occur more frequently in sickle cell disease than in sickle cell trait, often will present with hematuria.

Vermeulen et al. [10] retrospectively reviewed data on renal pathology from sub-Saharan Africa and noted that secondary glomerular diseases (49.3%) occurred more frequently than primary glomerular diseases (39.7%). The most frequent primary glomerular diseases were focal segmental glomerulosclerosis (29.6%), membranous glomerulonephritis and membrano-proliferative glomerulonephritis (18.1%). While lupus nephritis (31.0%) was the most frequent secondary glomerular disease, followed by HIV-associated nephropathy (HIVAN) (13.3%) and malignant hypertension (12.5%).

Urinary tract infections (UTI) are also highly prevalent in Africa. In a study in rural Nigeria, almost 40% of the 516 subjects studied had UTI. Females had a 3 to 17 fold increased risk of acquiring UTI, compared to their male counterpart, with Escherichia *coli* being the predominant causative organism [11].

3. Anatomic/Physiologic Characteristics in the Aging Kidney

With normal aging, structural and functional changes occur in many organ systems, even in the absence of any disease. The kidney is one of the most significantly affected organs. Both structural and functional changes occur in the aging kidney.

3.1. Age - Related Structural Changes

With aging, various structural changes occur in the glomeruli, glomerular basement membrane, tubule-interstitium as well as renal vasculature. Intrarenal vascular changes start with arterial intimal fibrosis and continue with arteriosclerosis and hyalinosis of small arteries. The arterial intima become less smooth and display endothelial dysfunction as part of the normal aging process. Sub-endothelial deposition of hyaline and collagen fibers results in intimal thickening and obliteration of afferent and efferent arterioles. Moreover, vascular stiffening and atrophy of the vascular media result in dysfunction of the autonomic vascular reflex. The major histological feature is nephrosclerosis, characterized by focal and global glomerulosclerosis, tubular atrophy and interstitial fibrosis [12]. The total number of functional nephrons decrease in the aging kidney [13]. In parallel with the decreasing total number of nephrons, hypertrophy of the remaining functional nephrons also occurs in older adults. As a result of these changes, total kidney volume decreases. In addition, radiologic changes such as kidney cysts, focal scars, increased cortical surface roughness and medullary volume, as well as decreased parenchymal thickness are more evident in the aging kidney [14]. Renal parenchymal cysts, usually considered as 'benign,' also become more common and more numerous in older adults.

3.2. Age-Related Changes in Renal Function

Functional changes accompany the structural damage in the kidneys. A combination of decreased functional glomeruli and structural glomerulosclerosis leads to a reduction in glomerular filtration rate (GFR) without a significant increase in the risk of end-stage kidney disease (ESRD) or mortality. The decrease in functioning nephrons puts older adults at higher risk for AKI. In older adults, mean GFR is approximately 50 to 80 ml/min depending on how it is measured or estimated. The 24-hour urine albumin excretion does not increase significantly with aging. Therefore, albuminuria may be a useful marker to differentiate normal aging and kidney disease.

With aging, the tubules also demonstrate functional changes with a general decrease in function. Conservation of sodium in response to an acute reduction of sodium intake is also impaired in the aging kidney. Similarly, the ability to rapidly excrete a large sodium load is also impaired. In addition, there is a decrease in both maximum urine diluting capacity because of medullary hypotonicity and the maximum urine concentrating ability [15]. Whereas, erythropoietin secretion, fractional excretion of calcium, magnesium, and phosphorus, and urinalysis are all normal in healthy older adults.

The older population also has an increased prevalence of many chronic diseases such as hypertension and diabetes mellitus. Age-related changes often overlap pathologic processes and several pathologic conditions of the kidneys might occur simultaneously in older adults. Therefore, it is sometimes difficult to distinguish between the changes expected in aging (physiologic changes) and those that arise from chronic disease (pathologic changes). Because of the high incidence of polypharmacy, drug-induced acute or chronic tubulointerstitial nephropathy is also seen more frequently in older adults.

4. Assessment of Renal Function in Older Adults

GFR is the primary tool to assess glomerular function. CKD stages are classified based on the GFR. Direct measurement of GFR is not available in most clinical settings and the optimal measurement of kidney function in older adults is not well established. Most laboratories report calculated GFR, which is usually estimated from serum creatinine value using the Modification of Diet in Renal Disease (MDRD) study equation or the 2009 Chronic Kidney Disease Epidemiology (CKD-EPI) equation [16]. Older adults show a poor correlation between serum creatinine and estimated GFR (eGFR). Furthermore, as the eGFR formulas utilize age, this may result in over diagnosis of CKD in older adults without overt CKD. Therefore, in the absence of abnormal albuminuria, a fixed threshold of eGFR (<60 ml/min/1.73 m^2), may not be appropriate for defining CKD in older adults. There have been calls for caution when defining older adults as having CKD if they have mild, stable reductions in GFR without any other evidence of kidney damage [17]. Despite the reduced level of GFR, serum creatinine levels usually remain relatively unchanged or increase only modestly over time with normal aging.

5. FLUID AND ELECTROLYTES IN OLDER ADULTS

Older adults are more vulnerable to changes in fluid and electrolyte homeostasis. Age-related decrease in the sensitivity to fluid volume and osmoreceptors leads to increased susceptibility to dehydration. Total body water declines by 10 to 15% with aging and can result in significant impairment in physical, visuomotor, psychomotor and cognitive function. The decline in total body water is mainly due to reductions in intracellular water and limited access to adequate fluid intake.

Electrolyte abnormalities, particularly hypo- or hypernatremia are common in older adults and are associated with high risk for morbidity and mortality. Hyponatremia is the most common electrolyte disorder in older adults. Syndrome of inappropriate ADH secretion, diuretic use and excessive administration of intravenous hypotonic fluids are major causes of hyponatremia. Impairment of diluting capacity contributes to thiazide associated hyponatremia, which is more common in the elderly population [18]. Hyperkalemia is also common in older adults due to hyporeninemic hypoaldosteronism with impaired ability to secrete potassium and excrete acid. In addition, hypomagnesemia occurs, often as a result of low dietary intake.

6. Clinical Kidney Problems in Older Adults

6.1. Chronic Kidney Disease

6.1.1. Prevalence of Chronic Kidney Disease in Older Adults

The Kidney Disease Improving Global Outcomes (KDIGO) practice guidelines define CKD as kidney damage (abnormal urinalysis, kidney imaging, or renal biopsy) or GFR <60 ml/min/1.73 m^2 for more than 3 months. The incidence and prevalence of CKD have increased in recent years in developed and developing countries. Approximately half of adults over 70 years of age have a measured or eGFR of less than 60 ml/min/1.73 m^2 [18]. CKD is also highly prevalent across Africa. Because of the lack of renal registries, there are no reliable statistics about the prevalence of CKD in the majority of African countries. Thus, the prevalence of CKD remains largely unknown, but, it may be much more frequent in Africa than in developed countries. In a recent meta-analysis, the overall prevalence was 15.8% for CKD stages 1-5 and 4.6% for CKD stages 3-5 in the general African population [19]. In Africa, like the rest of the world, the older population is increasing. However, unlike western countries, CKD affects mainly young adults in Africa [20].

6.1.2. Risk Factors for Chronic Kidney Disease in Older Adults

Advanced age is one of the strong predictors of CKD. But, CKD from aging alone does not, by itself, usually progress to ESRD. Hypertension is the most common cause of CKD in Africa. Other risk factors for the development of CKD include type 2 diabetes mellitus, use of non-steroidal anti-inflammatory drugs, obesity, dyslipidemia, hyperuricemia, infections, kidney stones, and auto-immune disorders. In Africa, the HIV epidemic is another relevant factor for the development of CKD. Sickle cell disease (SCD) which primarily affects black populations is also an important contributor to CKD in Africa, though majority of SCD patients have significantly limited life spans with most not living beyond the 5th decade [21].

6.2. Glomerular Diseases

Glomerular disease is common in Africa and is a major cause of ESRD. The patterns of the renal disease currently seen in older Africans is similar to those in other continents. Primary and secondary glomerular diseases can present in different forms in the older adults. Nephrotic syndrome is the most common indication for renal biopsy. Membranous nephropathy (MN) is reported as the most common type of primary glomerular disease in older adults [22]. Most cases of MN (80%) are idiopathic and 20% are secondary to solid organ tumors and drugs in older adults. Most patients with MN present with typical features of nephrotic syndrome (>85%), but a few present with asymptomatic proteinuria, often without hematuria [23].

A kidney biopsy is the most reliable tool to accurately diagnose the specific cause of glomerular disease. It not only distinguishes the different types of glomerular diseases but also determines the chances of recovery of kidney function. However, the decision to perform a kidney biopsy in older adults is not an easy one for clinicians, as co-morbidities, shorter life expectancy, and complications of renal biopsy are significant challenges [24].

It is also important to consider sudden decreases in GFR, the presence of proteinuria and active urinary sediment as evidence of renal glomerular disease other than the age-related reduction in GFR.

Conservative treatment should be considered in older patients with glomerular disease. These include salt restriction, smoking cessation, renin-angiotensin-aldosterone system blockers, statins, and anticoagulant agents. Immunosuppressive therapy should only be considered in cases with nephrotic range proteinuria, progressively declining renal functions and in patients with rapidly progressive glomerulonephritis [24].

6.3. Acute Kidney Injury (AKI) in Older Adults

AKI is more common in the older patients compared to younger patients. In older adults, the etiology of AKI is often multifactorial and sometimes iatrogenic. Like in other age groups, AKI in older adults may be due to pre-renal, renal and post-renal causes. Pre-renal causes are more commonly encountered in older adults with poor cardiac function and dehydration with resulting hypoperfusion. Renal causes include sepsis leading to acute tubular necrosis (ATN), and administration of nephrotoxic agents which may cause ATN or acute interstitial nephritis (AIN). In Africa, the common use of traditional medicines which are often nephrotoxic greatliy contributes to the development of AKI [25]. Furthermore, intrarenal causes include acute glomerulonephritis and AIN as a result of polypharmacy. Post renal causes of AKI is also commonly seen in older men with obstructive nephropathy, due to enlarged prostate from benign prostatic hypertrophy and prostate cancer.

While the diagnostic tools for AKI are similar across age groups, physicians tend to perform less renal biopsies for older adults with AKI, mainly because of risks associated with renal biopsies in that age group.

Management of AKI in older adults is similar to the younger patients. It requires careful monitoring of fluid and electrolyte balance, in addition to preventive strategies such as avoiding nephrotoxins, radiocontrast agents, and volume depletion [26]. Patients should be assessed for post-renal causes of AKI with urethral catheterization and/or ultrasonography. Though volume status assessment can be challenging in this population, volume status should be carefully evaluated to guide further management.

In patients with severe AKI, standard renal replacement therapy (RRT) with dialysis including slow continuous methods should be considered. In oldest old patients (85 years and above) with AKI requiring dialysis, the decision whether or not to proceed with dialysis can be difficult. Such patients frequently have multiple comorbidities and associated poor prognosis. Frank discussion with these patients and their families about prognosis would be warranted. Starting RRT in older adults raises the question of appropriateness of life sustaining measures such as dialysis and renal transplant in those of advanced age, in light of limited healthcare resources in several African countries. Physicians and family members are faced with the difficult decision of withholding or withdrawing these life sustaining measures particularly at the end of life. This decision often requires a multidisciplinary team, support for the patient and family, and honest discussions about prognosis and goals of medical care.

The prognosis of AKI in the older adults depends on its severity and on the underlying disease. Non-recovery of renal function after an AKI episode in the older adults is common due to their multiple risk factors stated above. Even if kidney function does recover after an episode of AKI, these patients will need to be monitored closely as they may develop CKD.

6.4. Systemic Diseases and Kidneys in Older Adults

6.4.1. Diabetic Kidney Disease

Diabetes mellitus is a common disease in older adults. Diabetic kidney disease (DKD) has become the leading cause of ESRD in developed countries. DKD is defined by persistent pathologic albuminuria (>30 mg of urinary albumin excretion in a 24-hour collection) and abnormal renal function. Similar to developed countries, the number of patients with CKD due to DKD has been increasing in Africa. The exact pathogenesis of DKD is complex and not completely understood. But, hemodynamic and metabolic factors play an important role in the pathogenesis of DKD. Limited studies are available regarding examining the diagnosis and prevalence of DKD in older adults. There may be a higher prevalence of unusual presentations of DKD (e.g., decreased GFR without albuminuria) in older adults [27]. Older patients represent a unique subset of the population who require more tailored therapy to avoid further co-morbidities. Current approaches emphasis individualizing therapy. The standard therapy of DKD is the triad of optimal glycemic control, blood pressure control with renin-angiotensin-aldosterone system (RAAS)-blockade as first-line agents, and optimization of traditional cardiovascular risk factors [28].

6.4.2. Hypertension

Blood pressure increases steadily with aging. High blood pressure is a major risk factor for cardiovascular disease. Hypertension is both a cause and a consequence of CKD. The prevalence of hypertension has increased substantially since 1990 and its prevalence in older adults is about two to four times higher than in younger adults in Africa. It is estimated that 57% of adults aged 50 years and above in Africa have hypertension [29]. Increasing obesity is one of the main causes of the increase in prevalence of hypertension in older adults. Older patients are more likely to be aware of their hypertension and more likely to be treated; however, less likely to achieve blood pressure control when compared with younger patients. The treatment and control rates of hypertension in older adults in Africa are generally lower than those in developed countries [30].

Treating hypertension can both reduce the rate of cardiovascular complications as well as slow the progression of CKD. Many aspects of hypertension diagnosis and treatment are similar in younger and older patients; however, many relevant issues require attention in treating hypertensive older patients. Lifestyle modifications (e.g., dietary salt restriction, weight loss in obese patients, smoking cessation) should be an initial recommendation. In the absence of an indication for a specific blood pressure medication, low-dose thiazide-type diuretic, angiotensin-converting enzyme (ACE) inhibitor/angiotensin II receptor blocker (ARBs), or long-acting calcium channel blocker can be started as initial monotherapy in older adults. Special attention should be paid to closely monitoring serum creatinine and potassium. Currently, there is no clear consensus regarding the optimal target of blood pressure in older frail patients, especially those 75 years and older with multiple co-morbidities. They may develop orthostatic hypotension, which could be aggravated by intensive antihypertensive therapy. In such situations, management of hypertension management is often tailored to specific patients.

6.4.3. Multiple Myeloma

Multiple myeloma (MM) is more prevalent in older adults. The clinical presentations range from relatively healthy asymptomatic patients to significant debility with anemia and pathologic fractures. The age-standardized incidence of MM tends to be the lowest in developing countries such as those in sub-Saharan Africa, with incidence rates as low as 0.4-0.9 per 100,000 of the population, which is a tenth of the incidence rates in developed countries. Risk factors for MM include pre-existing monoclonal gammopathy and autosomal genetic mutations. It is also thought that the low diagnostic capability in developing countries may be a reason for lower incidence rates in those countries [31].

Kidney involvement most often occurs due to primary amyloidosis (AL type), tubular toxic effects of light chain, cast formation, and/or plasma cell infiltration. Hypercalcemia, volume depletion, hyperuricemia, and nephrotoxic drugs may contribute to development of AKI in patients with MM. Chemotherapeutic options are determined according to patient stratification based on age, presence of co-morbidities and cytogenetic abnormalities. The prognosis of MM depends on a variety of paraproteins, stage of disease and type of chemotherapeutic regimen.

6.5. Urinary Tract Infections

Urinary tract infection (UTI) is one of the most common bacterial infections in older adults. Escherichia coli is the most common uropathogen. Predisposing factors for UTI include structural and functional abnormalities of the urinary tract, comorbid conditions, and invasive instrumentation/operations. Older, sicker, and less mobile patients are more susceptible to UTI. As in younger patients, the same algorithm is used for the diagnosis of UTI in older patients. Diagnosis can however, be challenging, as these patients are less likely to present with typical clinical symptoms such as dysuria, fever and may have less obvious clinical symptoms or symptoms that mimic other chronic conditions such as urinary frequency, malaise or delirium [32]. The clinical spectrum of UTI ranges from asymptomatic pyuria to severe sepsis. Treatment of uncomplicated UTI is similar to younger patients. Nitrofurantoin or trimethoprim-sulfamethoxazole is recommended for uncomplicated UTI, if local resistance rates do not exceed 20%. Acute pyelonephritis is treated with intravenous antibiotics with ampicillin and an aminoglycoside or a third-generation cephalosporin or a fluoroquinolone. Resistance to quinolones is high and they should only be used based on culture antibiotic susceptibility test. Prevention strategies for recurrent UTI should be considered.

6.6. Obstructive Nephropathy

Urinary tract obstruction is more commonly encountered in older adults. The obstruction can occur at any level of the urinary tract and lead to obstructive nephropathy (AKI or CKD). It may be acute or chronic, partial or complete, and unilateral or bilateral. In older males, the most common cause of lower urinary tract obstruction is benign prostatic hypertrophy or carcinoma. In older females, the most common cause of obstructive nephropathy is ureteral obstruction caused by pelvic malignancy. Urethral stricture disease, often secondary to trauma, may also cause infravesical obstruction in older patients. Upper urinary tract obstruction can be asymptomatic. Patients with slowly developing obstruction typically have no changes in the urinalysis. Urinary tract imaging should be included in the evaluation of individuals who present with impaired renal function.

6.7. Renovascular Disease in Older Adults

Renovascular diseases are encountered usually in patients with atherosclerotic disease and include two entities; renal artery stenosis (RAS) and microvascular diseases, which affect intrarenal arteries. Renovascular disease can cause both secondary hypertension and ischemic nephropathy in older adults. A patient with the clinical findings suggesting secondary hypertension should be investigated for RAS. Duplex Doppler ultrasonography, computed tomographic angiography, and magnetic resonance angiography can be used to diagnose RAS. The diagnostic gold standard for RAS is renal arteriography, which can be performed in older patients with relative benefit over the risk of procedure. The test of choice should be based on the presence or absence of renal insufficiency, local availability and clinical expertise with each technique. Medical therapy or percutaneous angioplasty with or without stent placement or surgical revascularization can be used in appropriate patients.

6.8. Hematuria in Older Adults

Malignant neoplasms of the urinary tract are more common causes of hematuria in older adults. Renal cell carcinomas (RCCs) are most commonly observed in the seventh decade. RCC is more aggressive in older patients, and treatment decisions can be difficult, especially in the setting of significant CKD where nephrectomy may lead to dialysis dependence [33]. However, increased use of renal biopsy to determine whether a mass lesion is malignant and localized resection of the mass or surveillance over time have become more common. These are usually the preferred approaches to RCC in patients with CKD.

6.9. Nephrotoxicity in Older Adults

Older adults with kidney disease are exceptionally susceptible to adverse effects from medications due to pharmacokinetic changes from aging, in additon to those due to kidney disease itself. Furthermore, medications are often prescribed to older adults with the assumption that a normal or nearly normal serum creatinine concentration is consistent with normal renal function, resulting in inappropriate medication dosing. It is critical not to rely solely on serum creatinine values for determination of dosages. Renal function of older adults is best estimated by the methods mentioned above as the Cockroft-Gault and the MDRD equations. Cystatin C-based equations have also been found to be accurate in estimating renal function, though this has not been well studied in the very old and are used to lesser degree in clinical practice. Another predisposing factor contributing to the nephrotoxicity in older patients with CKD is polypharmacy which is the result of multiple medications often prescribed by multiple physicians. This creates a great risk for drug-drug interactions that can be exacerbated when renal clearance is impaired. In Africa, the common use of traditional medicines remains a significant contributor to nephrotoxicity [25].

6.10. Renal Replacement Therapies and Conservative Therapy in Older Adults

Renal replacement therapies (RRT) include hemodialysis, peritoneal dialysis and renal transplantation. These modalities have relatively limited availability in Africa, particularly sub-Saharan Africa, compared to the other continents, mainly due to high poverty rates, shortage of qualified medical professionals and unavailability of adequate medical care [3, 33]. Of the three modalities, in-center hemodialysis in the most commonly utilized on the continent. These dialysis centers are usually available in tertiary institutions located in major cities. This, together with the high cost makes it inaccessible to majority of the population. In addition, health care costs in majority of countries in Africa are mainly borne by the patient through private pay. This often makes long term chronic hemodialysis unattainable, resulting in patients being under-dialyzed [34]. Chronic peritoneal dialysis has even less availability due to high costs of dialytic fluid, low levels of health literacy and possibly high rate of peritonitis. Kidney transplantation is the least available of the RRT modalities and are carried out in few countries in Africa such as South Africa, Egypt, Nigeria, Ghana and Mauritius. Few African countries such as South Africa and Mauritius provide healthcare coverage for RRT, for indigent patients who are eligible for kidney transplantation. Most of these transplants are from living donors, with few centers in South Africa utilizing deceased donors [3, 35]. Data in developing countries also indicate higher mortality in older kidney transplant patients, which is consistent with those in developed countries [35, 36].

Conservative therapy of ESRD which mainly involves symptomatic and comfort based treatments is favored by many older adults and there is some evidence that there is no significant difference in overall QOL scores in older adults undergoing RRT compared to those opting for conservative measures

[34, 37]. In African countries, where there is significant scarcity of health resources, a large number of older patients end up with conservative or no treatment for their ESRD, by default [35, 36]. In spite of this, there is growing awareness with institution of primary and secondary CKD prevention strategies across the continent, in addition to a focus on promoting public health education, increasing health literacy and screening high risk populations [3]. A number of these initiatives are still in infancy stages but show great promise in a continent grappling with many challenges.

In summary, recognizing the similarities and differences in the kidney diseases between patients in Africa and other developed countries is critical. Identifying the uniqueness of some of the etiology and pathogenesis of kidney diseases in Africa may help better manage these diseases and lead to better quality of life and survival in these patients.

REFERENCES

[1] Population Reference Bureau. (August 24, 2018). Average life expectancy* in Africa for those born in 2018, by gender and region (in years) [Graph]. In: *Statista*. Retrieved September 13, 2019, from https://www.statista.com/statistics/274511/life-expectancy-in-africa/.

[2] Arogundade FA, Hassan MO, Bolanle A. Omotoso BA, et al. Spectrum of kidney diseases in Africa: malaria, schistosomiasis, sickle cell disease, and toxins. *Clinical Nephrology*, Vol. 86. Suppl. 1/2016 (S53-S60).

[3] Naicker S. Burden of end-stage renal disease in sub-Saharan Africa. *Clin. Nephrol*. 2010;74 Suppl 1:S13-6.

[4] Marie P Halle, Christian Takongue, Andre P Kengne, Epidemiological profile of patients with end stage renal disease in a referral hospital in Cameroon. *BMC Nephrology* (2015) 16:59.

[5] Naicker S, Aboud O, Gharbi MB et al. Epidemiology of acute kidney injury in Africa. *Semin. Nephrol*. 2008 Jul; 28(4):348-53.

[6] Adibe MO, Ewelum PC, Amorha KC. Evaluation of drug-drug interactions among patients with chronic kidney disease in a South-Eastern Nigeria tertiary hospital: a retrospective study. *Pan. African Med. J.* 2017; 28:199.

[7] Adu D, Okyere P, Boima V, Matekole M, Osafo C. *Clin. Nephrol.* Community-acquired acute kidney injury in adults in Africa. 2016 Supplement 1;86 (2016)(13):48-52.

[8] Pereira J, Calleia E, Marne C, Borque A. Vesical schistosomiasis with terminal hematuria in sub-Saharan patients. *S. Afr. Med. J.* 2019 Jun 28; 109(7):486-492.

[9] Aeddula NR and Baradhi KM. *Sickle cell nephropathy.* StatPearls [Internet]. Treasure Island (FL): StatPearls Publishing; 2019 Mar 24.

[10] Vermeulen A, Menezes CN, Mashabane M, Butler OK, Mosiane P, Goetsch S, Naicker S. Patterns of renal disease: A 30-year renal biopsy study at Chris Hani Baragwanath Academic Hospital, Soweto, Johannesburg, South Africa. *S. Afr. Med. J.* 2019; 28;109(7):486-492.

[11] Oladeinde BH, Omoregie R, Olley M, Anunibe JA. Urinary tract infection in a rural community of Nigeria. *N. Am. J. Med. Sci.* 2011; 3(2):75-77. doi: 10.4297/najms.2011.375.

[12] Pannarale G, Carbone R, Del Mastro G, Gallo C, Gattullo V, Natalicchio L, et al. The aging kidney: structural changes. *J. Nephrol.* 2010; 23 Suppl. 15:S37-40.

[13] Rule AD, Amer H, Cornell LD, Taler SJ, Cosio FG, Kremers WK, et al. The association between age and nephrosclerosis on renal biopsy among healthy adults. *Ann. Intern. Med.* 2010; 152(9):561-7.

[14] Denic A, Glassock RJ, Rule AD. Structural and Functional Changes With the Aging Kidney. *Adv. Chronic Kidney Dis.* 2016; 23(1):19-28.

[15] Musso CG, Oreopoulos DG. Aging and physiological changes of the kidneys including changes in glomerular filtration rate. *Nephron. Physiol.* 2011; 119 Suppl. 1:p1-5.

[16] Levey AS, Stevens LA, Schmid CH, Zhang YL, Castro AF, Feldman HI, et al. A new equation to estimate glomerular filtration rate. *Ann. Intern. Med.* 2009; 150(9):604-12.

[17] Glassock RJ. Con: Thresholds to define chronic kidney disease should not be age dependent. *Nephrol. Dial. Transplant*. 2014; 29(4):774-9; discussion 9-82.

[18] Rodenburg EM, Hoorn EJ, Ruiter R, Lous JJ, Hofman A, Uitterlinden AG, et al. Thiazide-associated hyponatremia: a population-based study. *Am. J. Kidney Dis.* 2013; 62(1):67-72.

[19] Ebert N, Jakob O, Gaedeke J, van der Giet M, Kuhlmann MK, Martus P, et al. Prevalence of reduced kidney function and albuminuria in older adults: the Berlin Initiative Study. *Nephrol. Dial. Transplant.* 2017; 32(6):997-1005.

[20] Kaze AD, Ilori T, Jaar BG, Echouffo-Tcheugui JB. Burden of chronic kidney disease on the African continent: a systematic review and meta-analysis. *BMC Nephrol*. 2018; 19(1):125.

[21] Naicker S. End-stage renal disease in sub-Saharan Africa. *Kidney Int.* Suppl 2013; 3: 161-163.

[22] Powars DR, Chan LS, Hiti A, Ramicone E, Johnson C. Outcome of sickle cell anemia: a 4-decade observational study of 1056 patients. *Medicine* (Baltimore). 2005; 84: 363-376.

[23] Okpechi IG, Ayodele OE, Rayner BL, Swanepoel CR. Kidney disease in elderly South Africans. *Clin. Nephrol*. 2013; 79(4):269-76.

[24] Glassock RJ. An update on glomerular disease in the elderly. *Clin. Geriatr. Med*. 2013; 29(3):579-91.

[25] Sumnu A, Gursu M, Ozturk S. Primary glomerular diseases in the elderly. *World J. Nephrol*. 2015; 4(2):263-70.

[26] Luyckx VA, Steenkamp V, Rubel JR, Stewart MJ. Adverse effects associated with the use of South African traditional folk remedies. *Cent. Afr. J. Med*. 2004; 50: 46-51.

[27] Kidney Disease: Improving Global Outcomes (KDIGO) Acute Kidney Injury Work Group. KDIGO Clinical Practice Guideline for Acute Kidney Injury. *Kidney Int*. 2012; 2(Suppl):1-138.

[28] Ekinci EI, Jerums G, Skene A, Crammer P, Power D, Cheong KY, Panagiotopoulos S, McNeil K, Baker ST, Fioretto P, MacIsaac RJ. Renal structure in normoalbuminuric and albuminuric patients with

type 2 diabetes and impaired renal function. *Diabetes Care* 2013; 36(11):3620-3626.

[29] Abdel-Rahman EM, Alhamad T, Reeves WB, Awad AS. Management of Diabetic Nephropathy in the Elderly: Special Considerations. *J. Nephrol. Ther.* 2012; 2(5).

[30] Bosu WK, Reilly ST, Aheto JMK, Zucchelli E. Hypertension in older adults in Africa: A systematic review and meta-analysis. *PLoS One*. 2019; 14(4):e0214934.

[31] Cowan AJ, Allen C, Barac A, et al. Global Burden of Multiple Myeloma: A Systematic Analysis for the Global Burden of Disease Study 2016. *JAMA Oncol.* 2018; 4(9):1221-1227.

[32] Balogun SA, Philbrick JT. Delirium, a Symptom of UTI in the Elderly: Fact or Fable? A Systematic Review. *Can. Geriatr. J.* 2013; 17(1):22-26. Published 2013 Mar 5. doi: 10.5770/cgj.17.90.

[33] Roos FC, Thüroff JW. Kidney cancer: Treatment of clinically localized renal tumors in the elderly. *Nat. Rev. Urol.* 2011;11:595-596.

[34] Bamgboye EL. End-stage renal disease in sub-Sahara Africa. *Ethn. Dis.* 2006; 16 (Suppl): 2-5-9.

[35] Seow YY, Cheung YB, Qu LM et al. Trajectory of quality of life for poorprognosis stage 5D chronic kidney disease with and without dialysis. *Am. J. Nephrol.* 2013; 37:231-238.

[36] Moosa MR. Impact of age, gender and race on patient and graft survival following renal transplantation-developing country experience. *S. Afr. Med. J.* 2003 Sep; 93(9):689-95.

[37] Balogun SA, Balogun R, Philbrick J, Abdel-Rahman E. Quality of Life, Perceptions, and Health Satisfaction of Older Adults with End-Stage Renal Disease: A Systematic Review. *J. Am. Geriatr. Soc.* 2017 Apr; 65(4):777-785.

In: Care of the Older African Adult
Editor: Seki A. Balogun
ISBN: 978-1-53619-295-7

Chapter 4

PULMONARY DISORDERS IN OLDER ADULTS OF AFRICAN DESCENT

Seki A. Balogun*
Associate Professor,
Internal Medicine and Geriatric Medicine,
Division of General Medicine, Geriatrics and Palliative Care,
University of Virginia Health System, Charlottesville, Virginia, US

ABSTRACT

Older adults of African descent, as with other older adults are at significant risk and are generally susceptible to lung injury and resultant pulmonary diseases as a result of age-related changes to pulmonary function. Lung infections such as pneumonia, pulmonary tuberculosis (PTB) and non-infective lung conditions such as chronic obstructive pulmonary disease, asthma, interstitial lung disease are prevalent in the older population worldwide, including Africa. The advent of human immunodeficiency virus infection has also greatly increased the prevalence of pulmonary infections, including PTB, fungal lung infections, which in turn may lead to chronic interstitial lung diseases. Long term exposure to

* Corresponding Author's Email: sab2s@virginia.edu.

cigarette smoking and environmental toxins, as well as chronic conditions such as connective tissue diseases are also key risk factors for chronic lung disease, often with high morbidity and mortality. Pulmonary infections are discussed in the chapter on infectious diseases in this book. This chapter mainly focuses on exploring the prevalence, etiology, clinical presentations and management of common non-infective lung diseases namely asthma, chronic obstructive pulmonary disease and interstitial lung disease.

Keywords: chronic obstructive pulmonary disease, interstitial lung disease, asthma, idiopathic pulmonary fibrosis, pneumonia, pulmonary tuberculosis, pulmonary function test, spirometry, influenza vaccination, pneumococcal vaccination, ratio of forced expiratory volume in one second/forced vital capacity (FEV_1/FVC), 2019 coronavirus disease (COVID-19), environmental and occupational toxins

1. Introduction

Age related changes in pulmonary function make older adults more susceptible to pulmonary injury and development of pulmonary diseases such as lung infections (pneumonia, pulmonary tuberculosis), chronic obstructive pulmonary disease (COPD), asthma and interstitial lung diseases. COPD and pulmonary infections are two of the most common causes of death worldwide. In 2010, non-infectious chronic lung diseases such as asthma and COPD accounted for 3.7 million deaths worldwide, while pulmonary infections such as pulmonary tuberculosis and pneumonia accounted for 4.8 million deaths [1]. These pulmonary diseases are also prevalent in older adults worldwide, with variable prevalence rates depending on the country and region. Diseases with obstructive lung patterns tend to be more common and have prevalence rates of up to 70% in adults in Asia while in some countries in other parts of the world, it is much lower at about 4%. There is paucity of data from African countries on the prevalence of these non-infectious pulmonary diseases such as COPD, so the health burden in many of these countries is underestimated [2].

Pulmonary infections such as pulmonary tuberculosis (PTB) and pneumonia are also very prevalent in older adults, more so in developing countries. This has been further complicated by the human immunodeficiency virus (HIV) epidemic, with resultant high prevalence of PTB-HIV co-infection, ranging from 14% to 31% worldwide [3]. The 2019 severe acute respiratory syndrome coronavirus 2 (SARS-CoV-2) infection, also known as 2019 coronavirus disease (COVID-19) pandemic has also been devastating worldwide, with almost 2 million deaths, affecting predominantly older adults with attendant high mortality and morbidity. In United States alone, there are currently over 20 million cases with over 350,000 deaths. The majority of SARS-CoV-2 infections are in African Americans, Latino Americans and Native Americans, with death rates up to 2.7 times higher than Caucasians [4, 5]. Interestingly, the African continent appears to have a much lower prevalence of SARS-CoV-2 compared to other continents, with South Africa being the only African country in the top 10 countries with the highest prevalence in the worldwide [6]. These pulmonary infections are discussed in a subsequent chapter on infectious diseases in this book, so the focus of this chapter will mostly be on non-infective lung diseases: asthma, chronic obstructive pulmonary disease and interstitial lung disease.

2. Asthma

Asthma is common in older adults and is characterized by inflammation of the bronchioles with bronchospasm. Prevalence in older adults worldwide, range between 4-8%, with similar prevalence in developed countries as well as several parts of Africa [7-9]. Older asthmatic persons will often have a history of asthma in childhood which persists into adulthood and later life. There are, however, a smaller percentage of older adults who will present with asthma symptoms for the first time as adults, which may make the clinical diagnosis of asthma more difficult to recognize and differentiate from other chronic pulmonary diseases such as COPD.

Asthma symptoms may be triggered by external irritants such as tobacco use and other noxious substances, as well as medications such as beta blockers, aspirin, non-steroidal anti-inflammatory agents (NSAIDs). Asthmatic patients also tend to have a history of allergies to specific substances such as dogs, cats and mites, which may trigger asthma attacks with exposure. Comorbid conditions such as heart failure, hypertension and coronary heart disease are also common in asthmatic older persons. The presence of these conditions may complicate the clinical picture and management, leading to worse outcomes [10].

Cardinal symptoms of intermittent wheezing, chest tightness and cough occur in both younger and older asthmatic persons, though older persons may be less likely to complain of shortness of breath or chest tightness, which may reflect physical adaptation to this chronic disease or lower health expectations with aging as older adults tend to ascribe symptoms to normal aging. Other symptoms include those related to allergic rhinitis such as nasal congestion or discharge, sneezing, as well as presence of nasal polyps. The diagnosis of asthma is mainly based on the patient's history and symptoms, but is typically confirmed on pulmonary function testing with spirometry and bronchodilator reversibility response. Asthmatic patients will usually have airflow limitation with reduced ratio of forced expiratory volume in one second (FEV_1)/forced vital capacity (FVC) of less than 0.7. For older asthmatic persons, reference equations such as National Health and Nutrition Examination Survey (NHANES) III and Global Lung function Initiative (GLI), based on age, race and physical function may be utilized for age-appropriate FEV_1/FVC values [11]. Post bronchodilator response with increase in FEV_1 of more than 200 ml or greater than 12% is highly suggestive of asthma. Bronchoprovocation testing with a methacholine challenge may be helpful in those older persons with atypical presentation and normal spirometry.

Home peak flow monitoring may be useful for periodic lung function assessments but in older persons, compliance and proper use of these may be an issue. Allergen testing and serologic testing may also be useful, depending on availability. A chest radiograph may be used to exclude other lung pathology and is usually normal in asthmatic patients. Other imaging such as computed tomography (CT) is usually not necessary, particularly in developing nations with limited availability and resources.

With clinical management of asthma, classification based on severity of pulmonary impairment and exacerbation risk is usually recommended. According to guidelines from the National Asthma Education and Prevention Program Expert panel, there are four asthma severity classifications; intermittent, mild persistent, moderate persistent and severe [12]. Patient education on recognizing symptoms and signs of an asthmatic exacerbation, proper use of inhalers and avoiding exacerbation triggers (including smoking cessation) are key. Pharmacologic management includes short acting beta agonists (SABA) such as albuterol or levalbuterol for relief of acute asthma symptoms and inhaled glucocorticoids (such as fluticasone, beclomethasone), long acting beta agonists (LABA) such as salmeterol, formoterol for long term control of asthma symptoms. Medications are typically recommended in a stepwise approach, with SABA as initial therapeutic agent, often utilized as needed, for those with intermittent asthma symptoms and inhaled glucocorticoids and LABA as second and third therapeutic options, for those with mild persistent, moderate persistent and severe asthma. Combination glucocorticoid-LABA inhalers such as inhaled fluticasone propionate/salmeterol are also very useful but care must be taken to avoid high doses of inhaled LABA due to risk of cardiotoxicity. In addition, short courses of systemic glucocorticoids may be needed for severe asthma exacerbations. Chronic oral steroid use is usually only recommended in severe asthma, as a last resort, when all other medications have been fully optimized. It is important to note that chronic glucocorticoid use, whether oral or inhaled may decrease bone density and predispose to osteoporosis leading to increased risk of fractures, particularly in older adults. Osteoporosis screening with bone density measurements and prompt treatment is advisable in these cases. Other therapeutic agents such as anti-leukotriene medications, anti-IgE and anti-interleukin 5 therapy may beneficial in maintenance treatment for those with inadequately controlled asthma symptoms despite optimal use of above core medications, particularly those with moderate to severe eosinophilic asthma [12, 13].

As part of maintenance therapy, influenza and pneumococcal vaccinations, as well as the newly available vaccines against SARS-CoV-2 infection are recommended and are particularly important in this subgroup of older adults as they reduce the incidence of these pulmonary infections which tend to be more severe in asthmatic patients.

3. Chronic Obstructive Pulmonary Disease

Chronic obstructive pulmonary disease (COPD) is a common lung disorder with persistent symptoms and characteristic airflow limitation. The prevalence of COPD is almost 11% worldwide, with the highest prevalence in North and South America (13-15%), and the lowest in Asia (7.9-9.7%). The prevalence in Africa is reported to be about 11%, however there is a paucity of data in Africa, with an increase in COPD cases by over 100% between 1990 and 2010 [14]. Chronic exposure to cigarette smoke, whether passive or active is the major risk factor for COPD. Exposure to other occupational noxious substances such as biomass fumes, inorganic and organic dusts have also been found to play a significant role in the development of COPD [15].

There are two main subtypes of COPD namely chronic bronchitis and emphysema, with chronic productive cough and permanent structural destruction of air spaces being distinctive features of each subtype respectively. There is however, overlap in clinical symptoms and presentation of both subtypes. Interestingly, there may be overlap in clinical presentation of asthma patients and those with COPD as well, with some patients having both asthma and COPD concurrently.

In clinical assessments of COPD, eliciting a cigarette smoking history or history of exposure to toxic fumes is important. This should include the number of years of exposure and with cigarette smoking, the pack-year history, which is the pack(s) of cigarettes per day multiplied by the number of years of smoking. The smoking exposure history, as well as history of exposure to toxic gases often correlate with the severity of COPD [16].

These patients often present with symptoms of dyspnea and chronic productive cough. Exertional dyspnea may be one of the earliest symptoms though in older sedentary adults, this may be less common. Episodic wheezing and chest tightness may also occur uncommonly with COPD, which may make differentiating these patients from asthmatic patients difficult. Physical examination may range from normal to features of lung hyperinflation with distant breath and heart sounds, wheezes and crackles, depending on the severity of the disease. Patients with severe COPD may develop a 'barrel-shaped' chest with increased anteroposterior chest diameter [17]. COPD diagnosis is typically confirmed with spirometry showing irreversible airflow obstruction, unchanged post bronchodilator response with FEV_1/FVC ratio less 0.7.

Initial management of stable COPD is usually with inhaled bronchodilators, short acting beta agonists (such as albuterol and levalbuterol) and short acting anticholinergics (such as ipratropium bromide), to relieve intermittent symptoms as necessary. Combination beta agonist-anticholinergic inhalers may be preferable for ease of administration and maximal effect [18]. For more symptomatic COPD patients, use of long acting inhaled anticholinergics (LAMA) such as tiotropium or long acting inhaled beta agonist (LABA) such as salmeterol and formoterol is recommended. There is a possibility of increased cardiovascular adverse effects from use of LAMA and LABA, though there is also data on long term safety in the use of tiotropium, a commonly used LAMA. Careful consideration of patients' comorbid risk factors is important when prescribing these agents. Pulmonary rehabilitation is also an important non-pharmacological aspect of COPD and is recommended in conjunction with pharmacotherapy for symptomatic COPD patients, particularly those with limited exercise capacity. In addition, patients with severe COPD symptoms and hypoxemia (arterial oxygen less than 55 mm Hg or pulse oximetry of 88% or less) will require oxygen supplementation. Therapeutic regimen may be adjusted depending on the response to the different treatment modalities [16, 18, 19].

Vaccines against influenza and pneumococcal infections are also recommended for COPD patients due to their susceptibility to pulmonary infections and resultant poor outcomes.

4. Interstitial Lung Disease

Interstitial lung disease (ILD) refers to conditions with diffuse parenchymal lung pathology and could be idiopathic or secondary, due to infections or exposure to environmental toxic agents. Idiopathic ILD includes idiopathic interstitial pneumonias and cryptogenic organizing pneumonia. Secondary infectious causes typically occur in immunocompromised patients and these include fungal pneumonias such as coccidioidomycosis, pneumocystis jirovecii, viral and atypical bacterial pneumonias. Exposure to occupational or environmental hazards such as asbestos, beryllium, silicone is a common etiology of secondary ILD. Certain medications such as amiodarone and prior pulmonary irradiation also are associated with development of ILD. Connective tissue diseases such as rheumatoid arthritis, systemic lupus erythematosus, scleroderma may also have pulmonary complications and present with ILD. Certain types of ILD are more common in older adults such as idiopathic pulmonary fibrosis (IPF), which is typically diagnosed after age 50 years. The prevalence of ILD is also highly variable depending which type. The prevalence of IPF is estimated at 0.2-8.8 per 100,000, with increased incidence with advanced age [20, 21]. The prevalence of secondary ILD is often related to that of the underlying disease. For instance, in a South African cohort, forty percent of patients with systemic sclerosis were found to have ILD [22].

Clinical presentation of ILD is also dependent on the type. ILD due to infectious causes or connective tissue diseases tend to have a more acute to subacute presentation which may include fever, shortness of breath, cough and diffuse opacities on chest radiograph. These patients may also have extrapulmonary symptoms and signs of the underlying disease or condition, such as in connective tissue diseases. Idiopathic ILD such as IPF will usually have a chronic, more indolent clinical course with possible history of exposure to occupational or environmental toxins, chronic cough (usually nonproductive), progressive short of breath on exertion, fatigue and in older adults, there may be a gradual decline in ability to complete activities of daily living. Non-specific lung crackles may also be found on physical examination and clubbing of fingernails may be seen in advanced forms of IPF. Diagnosis is confirmed with pulmonary function test including spirometry, lung volumes and diffusing lung capacity for carbon monoxide (DLCO), showing a restrictive lung pattern with reduced lung volumes and DLCO. There may be a co-existing obstructive lung pattern if there is concomitant emphysema as can sometimes be found with IPF. Pulmonary imaging with chest radiograph or computed tomography (CT), where available, typically show lung parenchymal opacities. Diagnosis of ILD can often be made without surgical lung biopsy or bronchoscopy and the risks associated with these invasive procedures need to be considered, particularly in older adults [20].

Patients with ILD will often require specialty care, in conjunction with a pulmonologist. Treatment of ILD mainly involves the treatment of underlying disease, if present, as well as non-pharmacologic therapies including supplemental oxygen for those with hypoxemia (pulse oximetry 88% and less) and pulmonary rehabilitation. Primary pharmacologic therapies for ILD have been explored over the last few decades, current recommendations include oral steroid therapy and immunosuppressants such as azathioprine and mycophenolate. These are often associated with adverse effects including gastrointestinal disturbances and bone marrow suppression, as such, they are used mainly in moderate to severe disease. Other immunosuppressants (cyclophosphamide and rituximab) may also be considered for severe cases refractory to other therapies [23].

Treatment of comorbid conditions such as pulmonary hypertension, pulmonary embolism, gastroesophageal reflux disease, diabetes mellitus and ischemic heart disease, is also of great importance in patients' overall quality of life and wellbeing [24]. With advanced ILD, mechanical ventilation or palliative care services may need to be explored. The prognosis is quite poor in certain types of ILD such as IPF, with median survival after diagnosis, ranging from 8 years in older adults age 66-69 years to 2.5 years in those 80 years and above [21]. Lung transplantation may also be considered in advanced cases, though there may be very limited availability due to inadequate resources and skilled personnel in developing countries.

As with all chronic pulmonary diseases, vaccines against influenza, and pneumococcal infection are also recommended in patients with ILD.

REFERENCES

[1] Lozano R., Naghavi M., Foreman K., et al., Global and regional mortality from 235 causes of death for 20 age groups in 1990 and 2010: a systematic analysis for the Global Burden of Disease Study 2010. *Lancet* 2013; 380:2095-128.

[2] Burney P., Jithoo A., Kato B., Janson C., Mannino D., Nizankowska-Mogilnicka E., Studnicka M., Tan W., Bateman E., Koçabas A., Vollmer W. M., Gislason T., Marks G., Koul P. A., Harrabi I., Gnatiuc L., Buist S. Burden of Obstructive Lung Disease (BOLD) Study. Chronic obstructive pulmonary disease mortality and prevalence: the associations with smoking and poverty - a BOLD analysis. *Thorax*. 2014 May; 69(5):465-73.

[3] Gao J., Zheng P., Fu H. Prevalence of TB/HIV co-infection in countries except China: a systematic review and meta-analysis. *PLoS One*. 2013 May 31; 8(5):e64915.

[4] *The Color of Coronavirus: COVID-19 deaths by race and ethnicity in the United States*. Available at: https://www.apmresearchlab.org/covid/deaths-by-race. Accessed on December 31, 2020.

[5] *COVID-19 Coronavirus Pandemic*. Available at: https://www.worldometers.info/coronavirus/. Accessed December 31, 2020.

[6] Matta S., Chopra K. K., Arora V. K. Morbidity and mortality trends of Covid 19 in top 10 countries. *Indian J Tuberc*. 2020 Dec; 67(4S):S167-S172.

[7] de Roos E. W., Lahousse L., Verhamme K. M. C., Braunstahl G. J., Ikram M. A., In 't Veen JCCM, Stricker BHC, Brusselle GGO. Asthma and its comorbidities in middle-aged and older adults; the Rotterdam Study. *Respir Med.* 2018 Jun; 139:6-12.

[8] Obel K. B., Ntumba K. J. M., Kalambayi K. P., Zalagile A. P., Kinkodi K. D., Munogolo K. Z. Prevalence and determinants of asthma in adults in Kinshasa. *PLoS One.* 2017 May 2; 12(5):e0176875.

[9] Oraka E., Kim H. J., King M. E., Callahan D. B. Asthma prevalence among US elderly by age groups: age still matters. *J Asthma.* 2012 Aug; 49(6):593-9.

[10] Patel M. R., Janevic M. R., Heeringa S. G., Baptist A. P., Clark N. M. An examination of adverse asthma outcomes in U.S. Adults with multiple morbidities. *Ann Am Thorac Soc.* 2013 Oct; 10(5):426-31.

[11] Quanjer P. H., Stanojevic S., Cole T. J., Baur X., Hall G. L., Culver B. H., Enright P. L., Hankinson J. L., Ip M. S., Zheng J., Stocks J. ERS Global Lung Function Initiative. Multi-ethnic reference values for spirometry for the 3-95-yr age range: the global lung function 2012 equations. *Eur Respir J.* 2012 Dec; 40(6):1324-43.

[12] National Asthma Education and Prevention Program, Third Expert Panel on the Diagnosis and Management of Asthma. *Expert Panel Report 3: Guidelines for the Diagnosis and Management of Asthma.* Bethesda (MD): National Heart, Lung, and Blood Institute (US); 2007 Aug. Available from: https://www.ncbi.nlm.nih.gov/books/NBK7232/. Accessed on December 31st, 2020.

[13] Chotirmall S. H., Watts M., Branagan P., Donegan C. F., Moore A., McElvaney N. G. Diagnosis and management of asthma in older adults. *J Am Geriatr Soc.* 2009 May; 57(5):901-9.

[14] Adeloye D., Chua S., Lee C., Basquill C., Papana A., Theodoratou E., Nair H., Gasevic D., Sridhar D., Campbell H., Chan K. Y., Sheikh A., Rudan I. Global Health Epidemiology Reference Group (GHERG). Global and regional estimates of COPD prevalence: Systematic review and meta-analysis. *J Glob Health.* 2015 Dec; 5(2):020415.

[15] Tan W. C., Sin D. D., Bourbeau J., Hernandez P., Chapman K. R., Cowie R., FitzGerald J. M., Marciniuk D. D., Maltais F., Buist A. S.,

Road J., Hogg J. C., Kirby M., Coxson H., Hague C., Leipsic J., O'Donnell D. E., Aaron S. D. CanCOLD Collaborative Research Group. Characteristics of COPD in never-smokers and ever-smokers in the general population: results from the CanCOLD study. *Thorax.* 2015 Sep; 70(9):822-9.

[16] Qaseem A., Wilt T. J., Weinberger S. E., Hanania N. A., Criner G., van der Molen T., Marciniuk D. D., Denberg T., Schünemann H., Wedzicha W., MacDonald R., Shekelle P. American College of Physicians; American College of Chest Physicians; American Thoracic Society; European Respiratory Society. Diagnosis and management of stable chronic obstructive pulmonary disease: a clinical practice guideline update from the American College of Physicians, American College of Chest Physicians, American Thoracic Society, and European Respiratory Society. *Ann Intern Med.* 2011 Aug 2; 155(3):179-91.

[17] Badgett R. G., Tanaka D. J., Hunt D. K., Jelley M. J., Feinberg L. E., Steiner J. F., Petty T. L. Can moderate chronic obstructive pulmonary disease be diagnosed by historical and physical findings alone? *Am J Med.* 1993 Feb; 94(2):188-96.

[18] In chronic obstructive pulmonary disease, a combination of ipratropium and albuterol is more effective than either agent alone. An 85-day multicenter trial. COMBIVENT Inhalation Aerosol Study Group. *Chest.* 1994 May; 105(5):1411-9.

[19] Tashkin D. P., Celli B., Senn S., Burkhart D., Kesten S., Menjoge S., Decramer M. UPLIFT Study Investigators. A 4-year trial of tiotropium in chronic obstructive pulmonary disease. *N Engl J Med.* 2008 Oct 9; 359(15):1543-54.

[20] Sharif R. Overview of idiopathic pulmonary fibrosis (IPF) and evidence-based guidelines. *Am J Manag Care.* 2017 Jul; 23(11 Suppl): S176-S182.

[21] Kaunisto J., Salomaa E. R., Hodgson U., Kaarteenaho R., Myllärniemi M. Idiopathic pulmonary fibrosis - a systematic review on methodology for the collection of epidemiological data. *BMC Pulm Med.* 2013; 13:53.

[22] Ashmore P., Tikly M., Wong M., Ickinger C. Interstitial lung disease in South Africans with systemic sclerosis. *Rheumatol Int.* 2018 Apr; 38(4):657-662.

[23] Chartrand S., Swigris J. J., Stanchev L., Lee J. S., Brown K. K., Fischer A. Clinical features and natural history of interstitial pneumonia with autoimmune features: A single center experience. *Respir Med.* 2016 Oct; 119:150-154.

[24] Raghu G., Amatto V. C., Behr J., Stowasser S. Comorbidities in idiopathic pulmonary fibrosis patients: a systematic literature review. *Eur Respir J.* 2015; 46(4):1113-1130.

[25] World Health Organization. *Global Tuberculosis Report 2020.* Available at: https://apps.who.int/iris/bitstream/handle/10665/336069/9789240013131-eng.pdf. Accessed January 2nd, 2020.

In: Care of the Older African Adult
Editor: Seki A. Balogun
ISBN: 978-1-53619-295-7

Chapter 5

INFECTIOUS DISEASES IN OLDER AFRICAN ADULTS

Oluwatoyin Falusi Nwafor*
Professor of Medicine,
Division of Infectious Diseases,
Cook County Health, Chicago, IL, US
Rush University Medical Center, Chicago, IL, US

ABSTRACT

Infectious diseases are a significant cause of morbidity and mortality worldwide and especially among older adults. The impact of infectious diseases as a cause of mortality is especially high in Africa where there are high poverty rates and sub-optimal access to diagnostics and therapeutics. Acute and chronic infections cause significant morbidity as the natural aging-related waning of the immune system occurs. Infections in older adults may be misdiagnosed or diagnosed late due to a variety of reasons including atypical presentations and lack of classic symptoms in many. In addition, complications of antimicrobial therapy such as renal toxicity and significant drug-drug interactions are accentuated with older age.

* Corresponding Author's Email: Oluwatoyin_adeyemi@rush.edu.

A comprehensive understanding of common infections in the older African patient will empower physicians and other health care professionals to accurately and efficiently diagnose, manage and prevent these infections. In this chapter, we will review the impact of aging and a waning immune system on innate and adaptive immunity, infection risk and response to vaccination.

We will also review a few common infectious diseases affecting older adults in Africa. These include HIV infection, Tuberculosis, Urinary tract infections, Pneumonias, Influenza, COVID-19, and Skin/soft tissue infections.

Keywords: infections, mortality, immunology, aging, vaccination

1. Infectious Diseases in Older Adults in Africa

Globally, communicable (infectious) diseases are the leading cause of death. Of the 8.8 million deaths in Africa, infectious diseases accounted for 5 million deaths (56.0%) in 2016. Leading causes of death in this category were: lower respiratory tract infections, HIV/AIDS, diarrheal diseases, malaria, and tuberculosis [1-2]. Infectious diseases in Africa occur in high numbers through all age groups, however the extremes of age are particularly hard hit.

Antimicrobial resistance (AMR) is a global problem, but the scope and impact in Africa is poorly described in the literature. The widespread availability and access to antibiotics in the absence of prescriptions make the issue of AMR one of great importance. AMR impacts the management of common infections and can lead to increased morbidity and mortality in already stretched healthcare infrastructures in Africa. A recent review [3] described the current status of AMR in Africa in relation to common causes of infections and drugs recommended in WHO treatment guidelines. Of note, AMR data was not available for 42.6% of the countries in the African continent. The review also showed that the level of resistance to commonly prescribed antibiotics such as quinolones and trimethoprim-sulfamethoxazole was significant. This review highlighted the need to conserve the current arsenal of antibiotics and enhanced education around antimicrobial resistance.

2. The Aging Immune System and Risks for Infection

Older persons generally have greater susceptibility to infections than younger adults [4]. Multiple risk factors for increased infection include 1)impairment of natural barrier defenses: frailty, reduced gag reflexes, thinning skin, dry mucous membranes 2) medications such as steroids and other immunosuppressants 3) the presence of comorbidities such as diabetes and vascular disease, 4) poor nutritional status, 5) poorer antibody responses to vaccination, 6) residing in long term care facilities, 7) delays in diagnosis and therapy, 8) poor tolerance to invasive diagnostic and therapeutic procedures, 9) greater risk of nosocomial infections, 10) higher rates of adverse reactions to drugs, including antibiotics.

The immune response to infectious agents and other challenges is attenuated in an older individual, thus increasing morbidity and mortality in this population. Immunosenescence represents a recognized feature of aging. As age advances, disruption of both innate and adaptive arms of the immune system has been reported. In addition, older adults exhibit a continual production of inflammatory mediators and cytokines, also known as 'inflammaging [5-7].

The odds that an infectious disease is caused by diverse pathogens is higher among older adults than among younger adults. This point is illustrated by these two following examples. Urinary tract infections in older adults are mostly monomicrobial, however pathogens not only include E. coli, but also other gram-negative bacteria, such as Proteus species, Klebsiella species, Enterobacter species, Pseudomonas aeruginosa as well as Enterococcus species. In older adults with bacterial meningitis, pathogens like listeria monocytogenes and gram-negative bacilli need to be considered and treated empirically in addition to Streptococcus pneumoniae, the most common meningopathogen.

Several studies have shown that certain infections occur more often in older persons; morbidity and mortality from infections are also at least three times higher than they are among younger adults [8]. Infections such as tuberculosis, pneumonias, urinary tract infections, skin and soft tissue infections, infective endocarditis, bacterial meningitis, and herpes zoster have worse outcomes in older adults.

Due to the increased vulnerability to infections, physicians need to have a lower threshold to suspect infectious diseases so that appropriate diagnostics and therapeutics can be initiated in a timely manner even with atypical symptoms. Older patients with a recent history of hospitalization or residence in long-term care should be considered colonized with a broader range of organisms and have a higher risk of multi drug resistant infections [4].

3. Nuances in Clinical Presentation in Older Adults

Key indicators of disease severity such as fever or hypothermia, leukocytosis or leukopenia, laboratory parameters may be less marked or abnormal at baseline in older persons [9]. Older adults may also have a lower baseline body temperature and a temperature over 99F should be considered elevated. Fever may be absent in these patients and studies have indicated that as many as 25% of older patients do not mount a fever. Atypical clinical presentations such as acute confusion or delirium or a subacute course with weight loss, weakness, anorexia or urinary incontinence, can lead to delays in diagnosis treatment in the older population. It is important to note that all fevers are not infectious. Other causes of fever include rheumatologic diseases, cancer and medications. Of rheumatologic conditions causing fevers in older adults, temporal arteritis and polymyalgia rheumatica are the most common.

There are commonly used medications that can suppress the inflammatory or immune responses. These include analgesics and non-steroidal which many older adults take for chronic joint pain and other issues. Older patients are also more likely to be on antidepressants antihypertensives, sedatives, steroids and hypoglycemics which may affect the inflammatory responses to infections.

4. Antibiotics in Older Adults

Older patients are more likely to receive antibiotics especially when institutionalized or hospitalized. The distribution, absorption, metabolism and elimination (ADME) of antibiotics is affected by the changes with aging. Older adults are also more likely to have polypharmacy, increasing the risks of drug-drug interactions and adverse effects. Aging is associated with decline in renal function in many older adults, which is important in dosing of antibiotics. Certain drugs such as aminoglycosides are especially nephrotoxic and ototoxic with worse outcomes in older patients. Due to issues of cost, availability and activity against multi-drug resistant (MDR) bacteria, these aminoglycosides tend to be used more commonly in resource limited countries in Africa. The lack of steady, routine access to renal and drug level monitoring likely increase risk of toxicity from these agents. Steps in selecting antibiotics in older adults should include identifying the most likely site of infection, reviewing clinical and epidemiologic data including local antimicrobial resistance rates and the patients' underlying comorbid conditions [10]. Vitally important in older patients who are at a higher risk of suboptimal renal and hepatic functioning, is understanding the pharmacokinetics and pharmacodynamics of the antibiotics and considerations for toxicity and drug-drug interactions. Older age is also associated with worse outcomes in antibiotic related C. Difficile colitis.

5. VACCINATIONS IN OLDER ADULTS

In the face of declining immunity, prevention with vaccinations is important in maintaining the health of older adults. Vaccinations in older persons are helpful to prevent infections such as pneumococcal pneumonia, influenza and tetanus. In addition, vaccines also reduce hospitalizations and death from these conditions. Older adults have an impaired response and experts recommend supplemental doses, higher doses or use of newer protein/immune-conjugate vaccines as measures to improve immune responses. The influenza quadrivalent vaccine is more immunogenic and routinely recommended in those over age 65years.

Recommended vaccines for adults over age 65 years are 1) Influenza (inactivated) vaccine yearly; 2) Zoster (recombinant) vaccine; 3) Pneumococcal vaccine; 4) PCV 13 conjugate vaccine (if they have an additional immune compromising condition e.g., advanced HIV, s/p splenectomy) in addition to Tdap booster every 10 years [11]. Infrastructure put in place for vaccination needs to be simple and innovative including mobile delivery and home administration. Issues with the cold chain required for vaccines are barriers in many countries. Another barrier is that older adults may be less likely to seek routine preventive care outside of emergencies. The cost effectiveness of vaccination and increased awareness of vaccine preventable causes of death need to be emphasized. With limited access to diagnostics and supportive therapeutics in many parts of Africa, the role of vaccination and infection control measures in prevention cannot be overemphasized.

6. INFECTIONS IN LONG-TERM CARE SETTINGS

Many older adults who are institutionalized in long-term care facilities, such as nursing homes are frail. These patients are highly vulnerable to infections because of their frailty; and physical and cognitive disabilities. In Africa, these care settings are uncommon, but with urbanization and youth immigration, it is projected that caring for the older adults in these settings will continue to increase.

These closed and sometimes crowded environments favor spread of pathogens. Fever and infections are among the most common reasons that nursing home residents are hospitalized. About seventy percent of infections in this setting are caused by lower respiratory tract infections, urinary tract infections, and skin and soft tissue infections, including infected pressure ulcers. The staffing issues, lack of space to cohort infected and non- infected patients to minimize the spread infection contribute to the spread of nosocomial infections. Education around hand hygiene and other infection control measures, vaccination and prompt recognition of infections to prevent outbreaks is key in these settings.

7. Specific Infections in Older Adults

7.1. Tuberculosis

7.1.1. Specific Disease Characteristics in Africa

Tuberculosis is the leading cause of death worldwide from an infectious disease among adults. Mycobacterium Tuberculosis (MTB) infects about 1 in 3 people in the world with over 9 million new cases and 2 million deaths each year worldwide. In Africa, HIV and TB are leading causes of death, with the immunosuppression of HIV enhancing TB infection. It is estimated that up to 40% of AIDS deaths in Africa is from MTB. From WHO data, 12 countries account for 70% of the reported worldwide TB cases with three of the twelve being African countries (South Africa, Ethiopia and Kenya). The impact of under diagnosis and underreporting from other African countries is unknown, In the United States, most MTB cases are among foreign born individuals from Africa, Mexico and South East Asia [12, 13].

Tuberculosis is a significant cause of morbidity and mortality in the older adult. A high prevalence of latent TB infection occurs in people born or raised in Africa. With age and a waning immune system, reactivation of latent infection can occur. In addition, the use of steroids, other immunosuppressives, poor nutrition and infection with HIV increases the risk of reactivation. Many older Africans have had BCG vaccination and may falsely think this is the reason for a positive tuberculin skin test (TST). Unless BCG vaccination is recent, positive TSTs should not be attributed to BCG. QuantiFERON (QTF-G) antigen assay testing is a newer technology available for diagnosis, though may be limited in access in parts of Africa. When there is a high clinical suspicion of TB, negative diagnostics do not rule out TB infection in older adults. Older adults are more likely to be TST negative. Older adults may have delay in diagnoses and even with prompt diagnosis and treatment, tuberculosis infection after age 65 appears to be more frequently associated with death. Reasons for higher morbidity with older adults include general stress, poor health and nutrition, use of steroids, other immunosuppressive agents that compromise immune system and concurrent diabetes or malignancy or HIV coinfection. All of which increase the risk of mortality and morbidity.

7.1.2. Clinical Management

Symptoms of tuberculosis can be vague and sometimes asymptomatic in early disease. Symptoms include anorexia, weight loss, fatigue, fever and night sweats, and productive cough with or without hemoptysis. The triad of fever, cough and hemoptysis is not often seen in older adults with TB. Massive hemoptysis can occur from erosion of a pulmonary artery, Rasmussen aneurysm. Pleural involvement can present with chest pain which could mimic other conditions. Other presentations include oral ulcers, ocular tuberculosis, otitis media, abdominal TB, involvement of liver, kidney, and central nervous system. Physical examination findings are non-specific in the absence of pulmonary disease.

Diagnosis is by a combination of imaging and microbiology data in addition to physical examination findings. Imaging by simple chest x-ray could show cavitary disease. Classic upper lobe cavitation is less common in older adults as that requires a vigorous host response which is less often seen in this age group. Findings on imaging include a military pattern, consolidation, pleural effusions, scarring, adenopathy or a mix of any of these findings. Other findings include poorly resolving pneumonia, or mass lesions. Laboratory testing is usually non-specific and findings of anemia of chronic disease, lymphopenia are seen. Abnormal renal or liver tests could also herald disseminated TB infection. Urinalysis may show hematuria or sterile pyuria. Hyponatremia could be a sign of syndrome of inappropriate ADH secretion (SIADH) in patients with TB and can also occur as a result of Addison's disease or direct central nervous system (CNS) disease. The most commonly extrapulmonary reported sites of disease are the central nervous system, bone and joints with the axial skeleton more frequently involved. A TB diagnosis should prompt an HIV test in all cases.

Sputa for AFB stains and cultures are key for diagnosis and useful in treatment and prevention. Sputum induction is helpful as older adults may not be able to expectorate sputum. In many parts of the world, invasive mechanisms such as bronchoscopy and biopsies may not be readily available. Culture is the gold standard for detecting mycobacteria in clinical specimens. There are three types of culture media commonly used: Lowenstein Jenson (solid, egg based), Middlebrook 7H11(solid agar based) and Middlebrook 7H12 (liquid). Growth on liquid broth requires 1-3 weeks of incubation, while solid media require 3-8 weeks of incubation. Commercial automated liquid broths like the BACTEC system facilitate early detection. Newer technologies like the nucleic acid amplification assays allow for direct detection of MTB in clinical specimens. The sensitivity of these nucleic acid amplification tests (NAAT) is intermediate between acid fast staining and cultures. The results are highly specific at over 95%, however the sensitivity differs based on smear status. Sensitivity is 95% if smear is positive but drops to 40-75% if smear is negative. It is important to note that clinical suspicion for TB may be the only positive finding and treatment be initiated appropriately. Many patients with TB may not have access to testing, may have negative cultures and unless there is an alternate diagnosis, they should get treated for MTB. The sensitivity of NAAT is low in extrapulmonary TB.

Testing of MTB isolates for susceptibility is important to guide therapy. Rifampin (RMP) resistance is associated with poor outcomes and predicts multidrug resistant (MDR) TB. Newer assays to detect isoniazid (INH) and rifampin (Rif) resistance rapidly are increasingly available worldwide. Drug resistant TB is increasing and risk factors include, exposure to a person with known drug resistant TB, exposure to someone with prior treatment failure, travel in an area of high prevalence and exposure to a person with active TB who remains smear positive after 2 months of treatment. Drug resistance can be primary (due to acquisition of drug resistant MTB) or secondary (resistance developing while on treatment). Multidrug resistant (XDR) TB is rare with small outbreaks associated with high mortality described in Africa and Iran.

The standard regimen for pulmonary TB is for six months with the first two months of induction with four drugs and then continuation phase with two drugs for four months. Extrapulmonary TB requires longer duration of therapy and once susceptibility findings are available, therapy should be altered accordingly. Directly observed therapy (DOT) is important and may be more important in older adults to ensure compliance adherence and good outcomes. Poor adherence to therapy is a risk factor for development of drug resistant tuberculosis, making DOT an important part of therapy. Paradoxical response, an immune reconstitution inflammatory syndrome can happen during TB treatment and should be identified and managed appropriately. It is estimated in one study that up to 30% of HIV patients receiving therapy for TB and HIV develop paradoxical worsening which may require a short course of adjunctive anti-inflammatory including steroids in some cases [9].

7.2. Urinary Tract Infections

Urinary tract infections (UTIs) are common in older adults and more common in women than in men. It is estimated that asymptomatic bacteria occur in 5-10% of women over 70 years annually. Risk factors include prolonged immobility, indwelling catheters, outflow obstruction from an enlarged prostate, urinary retention or overflow from neurogenic bladder and comorbidities such as diabetes. In nursing home residents and hospitalized adults, the rates of bacteriuria in men and women approach 10-20%.

Asymptomatic bacteriuria in older adults does not require antibiotics as studies have shown no benefit of treatment. Symptomatic UTIs in older adults can be associated with significant morbidity and mortality, especially if associated with bacteremia. The usual causes of infection are similar to those in younger persons. In institutionalized older patients, two-thirds of UTIs are caused by Escherichia Coli and Proteus spp and a high prevalence of Klebsiella and pseudomonas spp. While most UTIs are monomicrobial, up to 20-25% can be polymicrobial in older adults. This is due to colonization, prior antibiotic use, bladder instrumentation and co-existing GI and GU flora with incontinence. Pyuria is not a reliable predictor of bacteria in many studies. The absence of pyuria in women is a strong predictor for absence of disease making the negative predictive value quite useful.

Symptomatic UTIs in older adults may not have the typical findings of urgency, dysuria or suprapubic pain and can present as altered mental status. Sudden changes in behavior, such as confusion or worsening of dementia, or the onset of urinary incontinence are common warning signs. Symptomatic UTIs should always be treated in older patients as they are associated with an increased mortality. Initial therapy for UTIs is usually to cover gram negative organisms, but because older adults have higher rates of polymicrobial infection, infections caused by gram positive organisms and resistant gram-negative organisms, it is important to obtain urinalysis and urine gram stains and culture prior to initiation of antimicrobial therapy [9, 14]. In patients with suspected upper tract infections, two sets of blood cultures should be obtained. In some cases, imaging with an ultrasound scan or CT scan may be performed. Many guidelines do not recommend routine imaging, though imaging should be obtained with unresolving fever or persistent back pain or continuing positive urine or blood cultures to evaluate for obstruction, stones or other nidus of infection such as perinephric abscess.

Therapy choice of a third -generation beta lactam or quinolone is a good one. In patients with instrumentation or known to be at high risk for resistance organisms, a carbapenem or aminoglycoside plus vancomycin is recommended pending culture results. The toxicity of aminoglycosides in older adults make these less attractive options, however due to low cost, they remain a viable option in many parts of the world including in Africa. The final therapy is guided by culture results and the absence of gram- positive organism on initial gram stain should lead to prompt discontinuation of vancomycin to avoid unnecessary exposure leading to antibiotic resistance. The duration of treatment depends on clinical response and site of infection, with upper tract infections treated for up to 2 weeks.

7.2.1. Prevention of UTIs in Older Adults

Studies evaluating the role of intravaginal estradiol in older women in preventing UTIs have been mixed. While a Cochrane review found that cranberry juice reduced the incidence of UTIs in women with recurrent UTIs, studies in the older adults have shown that cranberry juice decreases the rate of bacteriuria but not UTIs. Use of condom catheters are less likely to be associated with bacteriuria or UTIs compared with indwelling catheters. Acute cystitis is treated for 3 days in older women as the failure rates with the single dose therapy used in younger women are higher. Men should not be treated with the short course due to the potential for a prostatic focus of infection and relapse and are treated for 10-14 days. Chronic prostatitis requires a longer duration of treatment of at least 2-4 weeks and up to 6 weeks with an oral quinolone or trimethoprim-sulfamethoxazole being good choices, if susceptible.

7.3. Bacterial Pneumonia

Globally, pneumonia is the commonest infectious cause of death and the second leading cause of overall life years lost. In sub-Saharan Africa alone, lower respiratory tract infections account for 390,000 deaths in older children and adults each year. In the US, over 60% of adults age 65 years and older get admitted to hospitals due to pneumonia. Older adults are at greater risk for pneumonia for a variety of reasons, including changes in lung capacity, increased exposure to disease in community settings and increased susceptibility due to other conditions like diabetes, chronic obstructive pulmonary disease or cardiac disease. While pneumonias are classified as community acquired pneumonia (CAP), health care associated pneumonia (HCAP) or Ventilator associated pneumonia (VAP), we will focus on CAP in this review. Of note, both the incidence and mortality from HCAP and VAP are increased in older persons.

Community acquired pneumonias occur more frequently and are associated with higher morbidity and mortality in older adults compared with younger adults. Older patients hospitalized with pneumonias have longer lengths of stay and are more likely to require ICU stay. The three most common pathogens causing pneumonias are Streptococcus pneumoniae, Hemophilus influenzae, gram negative enteric bacilli and Staph aureus. In addition to bacterial causes, viruses such as RSV, Influenza, Human metapneumovirus and rhinoviruses can cause lower respiratory tract infections clinically similar to influenza [15].

7.3.1. Clinical Presentation

Classic symptoms like chills, cough and fever are less frequent in older adults, and pneumonia can present as confusion or delirium. Age is associated with a poorer outcome, higher morbidity and mortality. In a recent review [16] of adults in Malawi (median age 34 years), CAP in Malawi was highly associated with HIV. S. Pneumonia and M. Tuberculosis were most common identified pathogens. 32% had a viral etiology with influenza being most common. Enhanced vaccination to prevent infections or severity are needed in Africa. In addition, early detection and treatment of tuberculosis is essential as TB is associated with increased mortality. The access to supplemental oxygen to manage hypoxia remains critical in the setting of CAP. In most sub-Saharan African settings, laboratory diagnosis of TB has until recently relied on sputum smear microscopy that has poor sensitivity, particularly for HIV-associated TB. The World Health Organization has advocated an empirical "step-up" approach, whereby anti-tuberculous treatment is initiated for HIV-infected adults with features of severe respiratory infection and negative sputum smears who fail to improve after 3–5 days of antibacterial treatment.

Radiographic facilities are limited in most healthcare facilities in sub-Saharan Africa where the majority of community acquired pneumonia (CAP) patients are initially managed. The use of objective CAP severity assessment tools has been shown to improve the recognition of patients with severe CAP likely to require intensive care support or those who can be safely managed as outpatients. Current South African CAP guidelines recommend that CURB65 be used to inform sites of care and initial antimicrobial treatment. The CURB stands for Confusion, urea, respiratory rate, blood pressure and 65 years of age or older. However, it has been shown that indices may perform differently in different settings due to differences in demographics, pathogens and comorbidity profiles in populations included in validation studies.

7.3.2. Treatment

Treatment of CAP is usually empiric to cover routine pathogens listed above and clinicians should be aware of local susceptibility data. Guidelines on management of CAP are published and updated regularly [17]. A key aspect in reducing morbidity and mortality is education around prevention of pneumonias. This includes avoidance or quitting smoking, pulmonary toileting, use of incentive spirometry soon after surgery and pneumococcal vaccine.

7.4. Skin and Soft Tissue Infections

The thinning that occurs with an aging skin can impair the ability of the skin to provide a protective barrier to surrounding pathogens. Skin breakdown from pressure ulcers or excoriations from dry skin, viral infections like herpes zoster (shingles) or medication allergies can increase risk of invasive infections. Bacterial or fungal foot infections occur more commonly among older adults with chronic venous stasis, arterial or venous ulcers, diabetes. Depending on the site of infection, infections can be monomicrobial or polymicrobial. Drug-resistant infections like Methicillin-resistant Staphylococcus aureus (MRSA), gram negative infections and polymicrobial infections are more likely to occur in those with prior antibiotic exposure and residents of long-term care facilities.

Pressure ulcers are commonly called bedsores or decubitus ulcers and can occur when a person is bedridden or otherwise immobile, unconscious, or unable to sense pain. Frail older adults are especially prone to developing these ulcers which can be complicated by infection. Older persons with poor nutrition, diabetes and vascular issues are at higher risk. Commonly affected sites include the ischial and gluteal areas, heels and back of the head if completely bedridden. Not all pressure ulcers are infected or require antibiotics and signs of infection including drainage and odor can occur with bacterial colonization. Fever, leukocytosis, increasing pain and marked elevation of inflammatory markers are more suggestive of infection over colonization. Once deep tissue cultures are obtained, broad spectrum antibiotics to cover gram positives, gram negatives and anaerobes should be initiated with de-escalation based on culture results. Duration of therapy is based on extent of deep tissue or bone involvement, presence or absence of foreign materials, adequate debridement and ability to reverse the cause of the pressure ulcers [18]. In many cases, antibiotics are not curative and may lead to development of antimicrobial resistance. Antibiotics should be used judiciously and in conjunction with source control to enhance the efficacy.

Management of ulcers include removing pressure on the affected area and keeping the wound clean and protected with dressings. To manage infected ulcers, extensive debridement with removal of all the damaged, infected, or dead tissue is critical, in addition to antibiotics and enhancing nutrition. These ulcers can be prevented by inspecting the skin over bony protuberances for areas of redness. With dark skin this early sign may be missed. Other ways to prevent these include, keeping skin clean and dry, frequent turning and repositioning every 2 hours, having soft padding in wheelchairs and beds to reduce pressure. For healthcare providers and other caregivers, practicing good hygiene such as proper hand washing remains important.

7.5. HIV Immunodeficiency Virus

HIV/AIDS is a major public health concern and cause of death in many African countries with more than two-thirds of the total infected worldwide being Africans [19-20]. Comprehensive data on the prevalence and conditions of the older HIV-infected African adult is lacking. Over the past decade, the yearly number of deaths from HIV/AIDS in Africa has more than halved with earlier diagnosis and access to highly effective antiretroviral therapies. More than half of people living with HIV are aged 50 and older, and this number will continue to rise with modern anti-retroviral therapy. There are three distinct but overlapping groups of older adults with HIV- first, those diagnosed decades ago and now aging with HIV, a second group recently diagnosed with HIV and a third group recently infected with HIV. With increasing awareness and testing these groups continue to grow and with access to antiretroviral therapy, many adults living with HIV continue to get older. Many older adults are diagnosed late with HIV due to lack of testing, lack of awareness and presentation with non- specific symptoms such as fatigue, weakness, weight loss or anorexia which may be attributed to aging. HIV targets the immune system and as immunosuppression occurs, the host is at increased risk for opportunistic infections and cancers. Older adults are more likely to present with advanced AIDS and opportunistic infections.

The aging HIV patient presents unique and complex challenges that require multidisciplinary care. The overlapping impact of lifestyle, HIV viremia, HIV medications, inflammation, immune activation and illnesses of aging make the aging population one that requires special attention. Since HIV has become a more manageable chronic condition, the main determinants of overall health and quality of life are more likely to be related to the long-term consequences of chronic co-morbid illnesses and less from HIV virologic control or immunodeficiency. In older patients with HIV, a geriatric type syndrome may emerge at a younger age and the manifestations of the syndrome will depend on a myriad of things, including how many years they have lived with HIV rather than their actual age. The picture is different for an older patient who acquires HIV now after 50 years versus someone who is now 55 and has lived with the virus for over 25 years. Even in patients with well-controlled HIV, there is an increased risk for diabetes, cancer, cardiovascular disease, osteoporosis and pulmonary disease. While a consistently undetectable viral load will improve long term outcomes, it does not eliminate the risk of HIV-related and unrelated cancers; and other conditions. Studies have also suggested that the appearance of geriatric syndromes, such as frailty and cognitive impairment, are seen in people living with HIV (PLWH) at younger ages than their matched peers.

In addition, older PLWH often face loneliness, social isolation and stigmata that can make care difficult. Some patients experience isolation from their families and have minimal social support. Financial difficulties and poor nutrition are accentuated in these older PLWH which further contributes to the impaired quality of life reported. Polypharmacy, defined as the simultaneous use of five or more medications is another concern commonly seen in the older population, but especially in older PLWH. Anti-retroviral medications often have drug-drug interactions and cumulative adverse reactions. African adults with HIV may still be on older anti-retroviral medications with adverse reactions such as lipodystrophy, osteopenia or nephrotoxicity. Commonly used medications such as statins, narcotic and analgesics, psychotropic drugs and diuretics can potentially interact with HIV medications or lead to cognitive impairments, hypotension and falls. Polypharmacy also increases the risk of poor adherence thus increasing the risk for poor outcomes. The details of the comprehensive care of an HIV infected adult are beyond the scope of this chapter and are well updated in HIV management guidelines [21]. Special attention to the aging HIV adult are highlighted in the guidelines.

7.6. Influenza

Influenza is an important cause of morbidity and mortality worldwide. In the US, seasonal influenza is a significant cause of death, 90% of which occur in older adults over age 65 years. The burden of influenza in Africa is substantial and underappreciated. Chronic underlying medical conditions, advanced age, frailty, and weakened immunity in older adults, increase the risk of developing severe complications from influenza, such as pneumonia. Patients in a closed or crowded environment like nursing homes are at higher risk of getting infected.

The burden of influenza as a cause of morbidity and mortality in Africa is unknown. Data from sporadic studies suggest that influenza is prevalent in Africa and the disease may have considerable impact on morbidity and mortality on the continent [22]. In most settings, acute febrile cases are treated for malaria and rapid diagnostics to confirm influenza are not readily available. Newly published national estimates describe for the first time the burden of influenza in South Africa; nearly 10,000 deaths and 40,000 hospitalizations are due to influenza each year. Influenza vaccination is significantly underused in Africa. As of 2019, less than 10 countries in Africa had a national influenza vaccination program. In those countries, priorities have been given to those with higher risk for adverse outcomes including pregnant women, older adults, and those with underlying medical conditions such as HIV. In other parts of Africa, influenza vaccination is sporadic and only available in the private sector [23]. There are limited data on influenza vaccine efficacy in tropical Africa. The vaccine antibody response in an African population to a vaccine developed mainly for populations in certain geographical areas of the world is largely unknown [24].

7.6.1. Clinical Management

Chills, cough and fever are the common symptoms, though again, influenza may present with predominantly gastrointestinal and other symptoms in older adults. These non- specific symptoms are often attributed to more common endemic infections such as malaria and typhoid fever, especially in settings where seasonal influenza is underrecognized. The lack of readily available access to rapid diagnostics for influenza makes it difficult to test for and initiate treatment. Older age is a significant predictor of mortality mostly from complications such as pneumonia and sepsis. Treatment is with supportive care and rapid initiation of antivirals-oseltamivir or less often neuraminidase inhibitors to shorten duration of symptoms [9, 24]. Annual influenza vaccinations are usually recommended for older adults in order to prevent infection. While not listed as a significant cause of mortality in Africa, African patients residing outside of the continent in other climates remain at risk and should be offered vaccination. For recent immigrants or visitors who have never received influenza vaccination, it may be initially rejected but with proper education, it is likely to be accepted as standard of care. A raised awareness of influenza as a cause of febrile illnesses and pneumonia in African patients is essential for the clinical management of patients.

7.7. COVID-19 (Corona Virus Infectious Disease - 2019)

The COVID-19 pandemic of 2020 is still raging worldwide. As of November 2020, there have been over 61 million cases and 1.4 million deaths reported worldwide. Africa, a continent with over one billion, has had about 2.2 million cases and about 51,000 deaths [26]. The lower cases and lower case-fatality rates in Africa are likely multifactorial including more asymptomatic disease, younger population overall, temperature/ climate differences and adherence with public health messages. Of note, less than 5% (about 3%) of the population in Africa is over 65 years. Another driver of mortality which is not common in Africa are group homes/residential facilities and nursing homes. It is the norm in many African countries for people to return to their rural homes when they retire from employment in urban areas.

7.7.1. Clinical Management

Older adults are at high risk patients for developing COVID-19 severe illness with rapidly progressive clinical deterioration. A waning immune response and a cluster of comorbid conditions increase the rates of respiratory failure, multisystemic involvement and death. Studies have shown that advanced age is the most important predictor for mortality. While males and females have the same susceptibility to COVID-19, male patients may be more prone to dying independent of age [26-28].

Age-related decline in clearance of inhaled particles and a gradual decrease in number of ciliated cells in the airway support increases susceptibility to infection. SARS-CoV-2 uses its spike (S) protein particle to attach to human cells. Decrease of ACE2 activity exacerbates the severity of lung injuries and inflammatory lung diseases. The most common symptoms are fever, productive cough and shortness of breath; concomitant less common symptoms are runny nose, headache, and diarrhea. The Pneumonia Severity Index (PSI) score of the older group is higher when compared to the young and middle-aged group. Atypical presentation in older adults may include delirium, low-grade hyperpyrexia, and abdominal pain, complicating the diagnostic course.

Radiologic findings occur early and CT findings are present even with patients with no respiratory symptoms or signs. Access to imaging is limited in most parts of the developing world and there is heightened concern with the shortage of necessary PPE and isolation protocols. When available, typical findings on computed tomography (CT) include bilateral multilobar ground-glass opacification with a peripheral or posterior distribution, mainly in the lower lobes. Atypical findings of consolidation which may involve multiple lobes can be seen in older adults. Unknown is the long term sequelae of interstitial lung disease or chronic thromboembolic pulmonary embolism in these patients. Adults 60 years and older, those with preexisting medical conditions, especially heart disease, lung disease, diabetes or cancer are more likely to have severe coronavirus infection than other age groups. The diagnostics, therapeutics and vaccines for COVID-19 are rapidly evolving and text in this section will be outdated by the time of publication. Mainstay of treatment is supportive care, use of supplemental oxygen and adjunctive therapies such as Remdesivir (an antiviral), Dexamethasone in patients ill enough to receive oxygen, Monoclonal antibody therapies and a myriad of therapeutics in clinical trials. At the time of this writing, three vaccines have been approved to prevent COVID-19 with good safety profile and efficacy of 70-95% in studies (29-31). The efficacy of these vaccines in older adults and the duration of immunity is still largely unknown but older adults have been prioritized for vaccination as high-risk populations.

7.8. Miscellaneous Infections

Other infectious diseases in older adults not discussed in detail in this chapter are Infectious Endocarditis and Chronic Hepatitis B and Hepatitis C, as they are also discussed in other chapters in this book.

Infective endocarditis (IE) is a relatively uncommon infection worldwide but up to half of patients in studies of endocarditis are over age 60 years. Subacute IE is a cause of fever of undetermined origin and failure to thrive in older adults and should always be considered in the work up of these conditions. The increased risk is related to older age with preexisting cardiac disease and increasing prevalence of prosthetic heart valves in developing countries. IE is not commonly diagnosed in Africa and will not be discussed in detail in this chapter [32].

Other infections that are treatable include Hepatitis B and Hepatitis C. Treatment is to reduce complications such as cirrhosis, liver failure and hepatocellular cancer (HCC). Cure of hepatitis C is associated with a 70% reduction in morbidity and a 90% reduction in risk of liver decompensation (ref). While cure of hepatitis C is the goal, management of hepatitis B is viral suppression. HBVDNA levels are strongly associated with increased hepatocellular (HCC) risk and suppressing HBVDNA once treatment is indicated reduces this risk. There is also need for screening for HCC in patients with chronic HBV and chronic HCV and guidelines for these exist. The diagnosis, management of liver and non-liver related complications for Hepatitis B and Hepatitis C are beyond the scope of this chapter and are clearly summarized in the guidelines [33, 34].

References

[1] GBD 2015 Mortality and Causes of Death Collaborators. Global, regional, and national life expectancy, all-cause mortality, and cause specific mortality for 249 causes of death, 1980-2015: a systematic

analysis for the Global Burden of Disease Study 2015. *Lancet.* 2016 Oct 8; 388: 1459–1544.

[2] GBD 2015 LRI Collaborators. Estimates of the global, regional, and national morbidity, mortality, and aetiologies of lower respiratory tract infections in 195 countries: a systematic analysis for the Global Burden of Disease Study 2015. *Lancet Infect Dis.* 2017 Aug 23; 17: 1133–1161.

[3] Tadasse BT, Ashley EA, Ongarello S, et al. Antimicrobial resistance in Africa: a systematic review Tadesse et al. *BMC Infectious Disease*s. 2017 Sept 11; 17: 616.

[4] Ouslander JG. *Principles of geriatric medicine and gerontology.* 4th ed. McGraw-Hill; 1999: 303-331.

[5] Tummala MK, Taub DD, Ershler WB. Clinical immunology: immune senescence and the acquired immune deficiency of aging. In: Fillit HM, Rockwood K, Woodhouse K, eds. *Brocklehurst's Textbook of Geriatric Medicine and Gerontology.* 7th ed. Saunders/Elsevier; 2010: 82-90.

[6] Castle SC. Clinical relevance of age-related immune dysfunction. *Clin Infect Dis.* 2000 Sep 14; 31(2): 578-585.

[7] Montecino-Rodriguez E, Berent-Maoz B, Dorshkind K. Causes, consequences, and reversal of immune system aging. *J Clin Invest.* 2013 Mar 1; 123(3): 958–965.

[8] High KP. Infection in the elderly. In: Halter JB, Ouslander JG, Tinetti ME, et al, eds. *Hazzard's Geriatric Medicine and Gerontology*. 6th ed. McGraw-Hill; 2009:1508-1515.

[9] Bennett JE, Dolin R, Blaser MJ. *Mandell, Douglas, and Bennett's principles and practice of infectious diseases*. Elsevier/Saunders; 2015

[10] Bolon M, Weber SG. General principles of antimicrobial selection. In: Halter JB, Ouslander JG, Tinetti ME, et al, eds. *Hazzard's Geriatric Medicine and Gerontology*. 6th ed. McGraw-Hill; 2009:1518-1530.

[11] U.S. Department of Health and Human Services. Centers for Disease Control and Prevention. *Recommended Adult immunization Schedule for ages 19 years and older 2020*. Available at: https://www.cdc.gov/

vaccines/schedules/downloads/adult/adult-combined-schedule.pdf Accessed December 4th, 2020.

[12] Pai M, Behr M, Dowdy D, et al. Tuberculosis. *Nature Reviews Disease Primers.* 2016 Oct 27; doi: https://doi.org/10.1038/nrdp.2016.76.

[13] Furin J, Cox H, Pai M. Tuberculosis. *Lancet.* 2019 Apr 20; 393(10181): 1642–1656.

[14] Kang C, Kim J, Park DW, et al. Infect Chemother. Clinical Practice Guidelines for the Antibiotic Treatment of Community-Acquired Urinary Tract Infections. *Infect Chemother*. 2018 Mar; 50(1): 67–100.

[15] Fine MJ, Auble TE, Yealy DM, et al. A prediction rule to identify low-risk patients with community-acquired pneumonia. *N Engl J Med.* 1997 Jan 23; 336: 243–250.

[16] Aston SJ, Ho A, Jary H, et al. Etiology and Risk Factors for Mortality in an Adult Community-acquired Pneumonia Cohort in Malawi. *Am J Respir Crit Care Med*. 2019 Aug 1; 200(3): 359-369.

[17] Metlay JP, Waterer GW, Long AC, et al. Diagnosis and Treatment of Adults with Community-acquired Pneumonia. An Official Clinical Practice Guideline of the American Thoracic Society and Infectious Diseases Society of America. *Am J Respir Crit Care Med*. 2019 Oct 1; 200(7): 45-67.

[18] Stevens DL, Bisno AL, Chambers HF, et al. Practice guidelines for the diagnosis and management of skin and soft tissue infections: 2014 update by the Infectious Diseases Society of America. *Clinical Infectious Diseases.* 2014 Jul 15; 59(2): 10-52.

[19] Joel Negin J, Mills EJ, Barnighausen T. Aging with HIV in Africa: the challenges of living longer. *AIDS*. 2012 July 31; 26(01): S1–S5.

[20] World Health Organization. *Clinical Guidelines: Antiretroviral Therapy*. Available at: https://www.who.int/hiv/pub/arv/chapter4.pdf Accessed December 4th, 2020.

[21] Clinical Info HIV.gov. *Guidelines for the Use of Antiretroviral Agents in Adults and Adolescent living with HIV.* Available at: https://clinicalinfo.hiv.gov/en/guidelines/adult-and-adolescent-arv/whats-new-guidelines Accessed December 4th, 2020.

[22] Yazdanbakhsh M, Kremsner PG. Influenza in Africa. *PLoS Med.* 2009 Dec 15; 6(12): doi:10.1371/ journal.pmed.1000182.

[23] Centers for Disease Control and Prevention. Global Health –South Africa. Influenza Program. Available at: https://www.cdc.gov/ globalhealth/countries/southafrica/what/influenza.htm. Accessed December 4th, 2020.

[24] Lindsey BB, Armitage EP, Kampmann B, et al. The efficacy, effectiveness, and immunogenicity of influenza vaccines in Africa: a systematic review. *Lancet Infect Dis*. 2019 Apr 1; 19(4): 110-119.

[25] McMorrow ML, Tempia S, Walaza S, et al. Prioritization of risk groups for influenza vaccination in resource limited settings – A case study from South Africa. *Vaccine.* 2019 Jan 3; 37(1): 25-33.

[26] Worldometer. *COVID-19 Coronavirus Pandemic*. Available at: https://www.worldometers.info/coronavirus/ Accessed December 4th, 2020.

[27] Perrotta F, Corbi G, Mazzeo G, et al. COVID-19 and the elderly: insights into pathogenesis and clinical decision-making. *Aging Clinical and Experimental Research*. 2020 Jun 16; 32: 1599-1608.

[28] Guo T, Shen Q, Guo W, et al. Clinical characteristics of elderly patients with COVID-19 in Hunan Province, China: a multicenter, retrospective study. *Gerontology.* 2020; 66: 467-475.

[29] Polack FP, Thomas SJ, Kitchin N, Absalon J, Gurtman A et al. Safety and Efficacy of the BNT162b2 mRNA Covid-19 Vaccine. *N Engl J Med.* 2020 Dec 31;383(27):2603-2615.

[30] Baden LR, El Sahly HM, Essink B, Kotloff K, Frey S et al. Efficacy and Safety of the mRNA-1273 SARS-CoV-2 Vaccine. *N Engl J Med.* 2020 Dec 30. doi: 10.1056/NEJMoa2035389. Epub ahead of print.

[31] Voysey M, Clemens SAC, Madhi SA, Weckx LY, Folegatti PM, et al. Oxford COVID Vaccine Trial Group. Safety and efficacy of the ChAdOx1 nCoV-19 vaccine (AZD1222) against SARS-CoV-2: an interim analysis of four randomized controlled trials in Brazil, South Africa, and the UK. *Lancet*. 2020 Dec 8: S0140-6736(20)32661-1.

[32] Abdulhak AAB, Baddour LM, Erwin PJ, et al. Global and Regional Burden of Infective Endocarditis. *Glob Heart.* 2014 Mar; 9(1): 131-143.

[33] AASLD/IDSA HCV Guidance: Recommendations for Testing, *Managing and Treating Hepatitis C.* Available at: https://www.hcvguidelines.org/ Accessed December 4th, 2020.

[34] Norah A. Terrault NA, Lok A S, McMahon BJ et al. Update on Prevention, Diagnosis, and Treatment of Chronic Hepatitis B: AASLD 2018 Hepatitis B Guidance. *Hepatology* 2018 (4):1560-1599.

In: Care of the Older African Adult
Editor: Seki A. Balogun
ISBN: 978-1-53619-295-7

Chapter 6

ONCOLOGIC/HEMATOLOGIC DISEASES IN OLDER AFRICAN ADULTS

Alwin Jeyakumar*
Professor, Internal Medicine, Division of Medical Oncology,
Dalhousie University, Halifax, NS, Canada

ABSTRACT

Globally, cancer remains a major public health and economic burden. There were over 18 million cases in 2018, with an estimated 29 million cases by 2040 due to aging and population growth. One in four men and one in five women develop the disease, and one in eight men and one in eleven women will die from it. There is also an increasing population of people living with cancer; in 2018, almost 44 million were diagnosed in the previous five years [1].

This disease affects older African adults all over the world and in general, their care would be considered less than optimal with multiple areas for improvement. There are major differences in disease type and expectations depending on where older African adults live.

Cancer kills the most people in poorer regions of the world. In developed countries, lower smoking rates, personalized medicine, more screening, better diagnostics, and treatments are reducing cancer rates and improving survival. Much of that progress is not reaching sub-Saharan

* Corresponding Author's Email: alwin.jeyakumar@nshealth.ca

Africa (SSA). Cancer deaths in SSA increased 45 percent since 2000 where it now kills more than a half a million people each year [2].

Keywords: Sub-Saharan Africa, African Americans, Caucasians, cancer, breast, prostate, colorectal, lung, cervical, hepatocellular, sickle cell disease, control and prevention, palliative care

1. Introduction

In 2018, an estimated 752,000 new cancer cases (four percent of the global total) and 506,000 cancer deaths occurred in SSA. While the overall cancer burden in the region is dominated by breast, cervical and prostate cancers, the cancer profile in SSA is diverse. The most common cancers (incidence) in men include prostate (69,000), liver (24,000) and Kaposi sarcoma (20,000). Breast (115,000) and cervical cancers (112,000) are the most frequently diagnosed cancers in women [3]. Lung cancer is a high cause of mortality in SSA men.

Cancer is an increasing problem in Africa because of aging and growth of the population as well as increasing prevalence of risk factors associated with economic transition (including smoking, alcohol, obesity, physical inactivity and reproductive behaviors) and certain infectious agents of importance in cancer etiology such as HIV [4].

Reviewing the African American population in the United States, where there is better record keeping, they bear a disproportionate share of the United States cancer burden, having the highest death rate and the lowest survival rate of any racial or ethnic group for most cancers. In 2019, there were over 200,000 new cases of cancer and 73,000 deaths in this sub-group. Prostate cancer is the most commonly diagnosed cancer in black men, and breast cancer in black women, each accounting for nearly one third of cancers diagnosed in each sex. Cancers of the lung and colorectum are the second and third most commonly diagnosed cancers, in both men and women. Together, the four most common cancers (breast, prostate, colorectal and lung) account for 54 percent of all cancer cases in African Americans [5].

Older adults are defined as those who are over 65 years of age. In the next several sections we will be reviewing care of common cancers and sickle cell disease in African adults in North America and Africa with a focus on older adults.

It is noteworthy that when deciding on an individual patient management plan; performance status and informed patient wishes should be used as the ultimate determinant for patient care. Performance status is determined by patient characteristics including comorbidities and not just age alone.

2. Breast Cancer (BC)

Globally, BC is the most frequently diagnosed cancer and the leading cause of cancer death in women. In countries with established breast cancer screening programs, most patients present due to an abnormal mammogram. About 15 percent of women are diagnosed with BC due to the presence of a breast mass that is not detected on mammogram. In the developed countries, BC mortality rates have been decreasing due to improved BC screening and improvements in adjuvant therapy. BC should be treated with a multidisciplinary approach involving surgical oncology, radiation oncology and medical oncology, which has been associated with a reduction in BC mortality [6].

In North America, black women and white women get BC at about the same rate, but black women die from BC at a higher rate than white women. Reasons include earlier stage at time of diagnosis in white women and more triple-negative BC in black women which is a more aggressive BC subtype [7]. Different concerns exist in Africa where the population is predominantly young, hence BC patients tend to be young and the pattern of BC that presents to practitioners in Africa is more aggressive. Also, implementation of methods of effective early detection, effective and low-cost, low-tech treatment of early onset BC, and management of the social, economic and psychological sequelae of the disease are required [8].

Early stage BC includes clinical stage I, IIA, IIB (T2N1 subtype). Patients with IIB (T3N0 subtype) and stage IIIA to IIIC disease are considered locally advanced while 5 percent of patients present with distant metastases (stage IV). Patients with early-stage BC are treated initially with surgery. Surgical approach to the primary tumor depends on the size of the tumor, whether or not multifocal disease is present, and the size of the breast. Options include breast-conserving therapy (plus radiation therapy [XRT]) or mastectomy; both approaches result in equivalent cancer-specific outcomes.

The surgical approach to regional nodes depends on clinical status of the axilla; in patients with clinically suspicious axillary nodes, a preoperative work-up including ultrasound plus lymph node biopsy helps determine best surgical approach; If lymph node biopsy is positive and patient proceeds directly to surgery, an axillary lymph node dissection (ALND) should be performed. If the lymph node biopsy is negative, a sentinel lymph node biopsy (SLNB) at the time of surgery is performed. Patients who present with clinically negative axilla do not require a preoperative work-up; these patients undergo an SLNB at time of definitive breast surgery. Patients who have <3 pathologically involved sentinel nodes by SLNB do not require an ALND. Whether or not patients with ≥ 3 pathologically involved sentinel nodes undergo an ALND is determined on an individualized basis, reviewing other tumor risk factors, patient's performance status and comorbidities.

Tumor characteristics are used to select adjuvant treatment for patients with BC. Patients with hormone receptor-positive BC should be offered adjuvant endocrine therapy. Adjuvant chemotherapy recommendations in these patients requires a risk-stratified approach that considers patient and tumor characteristics. For patients with estrogen receptor (ER), progesterone receptor, and human epidermal growth factor receptor 2 (HER2) negative disease (known as triple-negative BC), adjuvant chemotherapy is offered if the tumor size is >0.5 cm. Patients with HER2 positive BC >1 cm in size are offered a combination of chemotherapy plus HER2 directed therapy.

Following chemotherapy, patients with ER-positive disease should also be offered adjuvant endocrine therapy.

Most patients with locally advanced BC and some with earlier-stage BC (particularly if HER2 positive or triple negative) are offered neoadjuvant systemic therapy rather than proceeding with surgery first.

Following breast-conserving surgery (with or without neoadjuvant systemic therapy), all patients should undergo adjuvant XRT to maximize locoregional control.

For older or poor performance patients due to medical comorbidities with estrogen receptor-positive BC, in whom surgery is not an option or life expectancy is limited, primary hormonal treatment with either tamoxifen or an aromatase inhibitor without surgery or XRT can be used.

On treatment completion, components of BC survivors care are cancer surveillance, adherence with treatment, lifestyle recommendations, treatment of medical and psychosocial consequences of cancer and its therapy, and care coordination between specialists and primary care providers. The majority of BC recurrences occur within the first 5 years of diagnosis, particularly with hormone receptor-negative disease.

Metastatic BC (MBC) is incurable, however meaningful improvements in survival have been seen with the introduction of newer systemic therapies. Median overall survival is now over three years, with a range from a few months to many years [9]. The goals of systemic treatment for MBC are prolongation of survival, alleviation of symptoms, and maintenance or improvement in quality of life. Given importance of hormone receptor and HER2 status in selecting treatment, where possible, hormone receptor and HER2 testing should be repeated upon diagnosis of MBC, in case there is discordance in expression between the primary site and metastases.

For most patients with hormone-positive MBC, endocrine therapy is recommended with or without targeted treatments rather than chemotherapy. If chemotherapy is needed, single-agent chemotherapy used in sequence, is preferable to combination chemotherapy since this is more likely to induce palliation with fewer side effects, and no studies have demonstrated an overall benefit for combination chemotherapy as long as drugs are available in sequence. Combination chemotherapy may be preferable for select patients with rapidly progressive disease. For patients with HER2 positive MBC, incorporate HER2 directed therapy with first-line treatment. Careful assessment of response to therapy using history and physical examination, radiographic imaging, and/or serum tumor markers will assist in decisions for treatment continuation and selection of subsequent treatments.

3. Prostate Cancer (PC)

PC is the most common cancer in men worldwide. In North America, 11 percent of men are diagnosed with PC over their lifetime, with the incidence rising with age. Overall 5 year survival rate is 98 percent and PC rarely presents with clinical symptoms. Uncommonly, PC may present with nonspecific urinary symptoms, hematuria, or hematospermia; more commonly, these are due to nonmalignant conditions. PC is suspected in patients who have an elevation of prostate-specific antigen (PSA) or an abnormal digital rectal examination (DRE). Although DRE is not recommended for screening; if performed, asymmetry, nodularity or induration raise suspicion for PC. The risk for PC increases as PSA level rises, although there is no specific numerical threshold that accurately determines the presence of PC. PSA changes over time are helpful in determining cancer risk. Investigation should follow shared decision-making with patients who have a life expectancy of at least 10 years. Diagnosis of PC requires tissue obtained by biopsy with imaging guidance. If a patient has significant comorbidities that limit life expectancy, further evaluation for asymptomatic PC is not warranted.

African American men both get and die from PC at a higher rate. The reasons for this are complex and unclear; in addition to differences in tumor biology, the higher risk may be tied to disparities in environment and behavior. Disparities in outcome could be affected by differences in when the cancer is diagnosed and how the men are treated after diagnosis [10]. African men suffer disproportionately from PC compared to men from other parts of the world. However, it is still quite difficult to accurately describe the burden of PC in Africa due to poor cancer registration systems [11].

Once diagnosis is established, management plan depends on pretreatment assessment of the risk of recurrence combined with patient age, life expectancy, overall performance status, presence or absence of symptoms, and patient wishes. Key factors in this assessment include clinical staging of the extent of disease, the pretreatment PSA, Gleason score in biopsy and imaging. With this information, patients are divided into several categories, which provide the basis for treatment decisions:

Clinically localized, very low-risk PC: Active surveillance, with serial monitoring and initiation of definitive treatment if there is evidence of progression, is a preferred care option for most men with very low-risk disease.

Clinically localized, low-risk PC: For men with low-risk PC and a life expectancy greater than 10 years, definitive therapy (radical prostatectomy, brachytherapy, or external beam XRT) or active surveillance are all options.

Clinically localized, intermediate-risk PC: Patients here are divided into favorable and unfavorable subsets based on the percent of positive biopsy cores and specific Gleason score or grade group. XRT and radical prostatectomy are both appropriate options for men with intermediate-risk disease. Active surveillance is an option for those with favorable intermediate-risk disease, but patients should be informed that this comes with a higher risk of developing metastases compared with definitive treatment.

Clinically localized, high-risk PC: Standard treatment options here include XRT using external beam combined with brachytherapy and androgen deprivation therapy (ADT), or radical prostatectomy.

Locally advanced and very high-risk PC: Tumors with seminal vesicle involvement (T3b), tumor fixation (T4), or invasion of adjacent organs (T4), as well as PC with a primary Gleason pattern of 5 or with four or more cores with a biopsy grade group of 4 and 5 (Gleason score 8 to 10) are classified as very high risk. Treatment options include external beam XRT, with or without brachytherapy, and long-term ADT. Radical prostatectomy with extended lymph node dissection is also an option for younger individuals.

Lymph node involvement: Clinical lymph node involvement is stage IV (metastatic) disease. These patients are treated with definitive XRT plus ADT. For young men with minimal regional lymphatic spread, radical prostatectomy as part of a combination strategy that includes postoperative ADT and/or XRT is an option.

Disseminated disease: These are stage IV disease; initial approach focuses on ADT, which can be combined with docetaxel chemotherapy.

High-grade, low-PSA PC: High-grade (Gleason score 8 to 10) PC with a low PSA comprise a distinct but uncommon subset that includes small cell and large cell prostatic neuroendocrine carcinomas. In patients with localized disease, treatment is similar to patients with high-risk disease. In patients with metastatic disease, there is an increased role for chemotherapy using regimens similar to those used for small cell lung carcinoma.

The prognosis for most men with PC is excellent. Due to a combination of older age at diagnosis, early detection, effective treatments, and a protracted clinical course, PC survivors have a higher risk of death from non-cancer causes than from the disease itself.

4. Colorectal Cancer (CRC)

CRC is a common disease and accounts for more than 10 percent of cancers globally. 70 percent of cases arise in the colon and 30 percent in the rectum. Patients with CRC usually present with suspicious symptoms and/or signs (change in bowel habits, bleeding, rectal or abdominal mass, iron deficiency anemia, abdominal pain), asymptomatic discovered by routine screening, or emergency admission with intestinal obstruction, peritonitis, or acute gastrointestinal bleed.

African Americans have the highest incidence and mortality rates of CRC of any ethnic group in the United States. Although some of these disparities can be explained by differences in access to care, cancer screening, and other socioeconomic factors, disparities remain after adjustment for these factors [12]. The incidence of CRC in SSA has been looked at, however few health services in SSA are equipped to provide timely diagnosis and treatment of cancer. In addition, data collection systems are weak, likely underestimating the burden of disease [13].

In developed countries, with increasing uptake of CRC screening, more cases are being diagnosed at an asymptomatic stage, still most CRCs are diagnosed after the onset of symptoms. A change in bowel habits is a more common presenting symptom for left-sided as compared with right-sided cancers. Hematochezia is more likely with rectal than colon cancers, and occult colonic bleeding is more common with cecal and ascending colon cancers. One in five patients with CRC presents with metastatic disease; the most common metastatic sites are the regional lymph nodes, liver, lungs, and peritoneum. A positive fecal occult blood test has a much higher predictive value for CRC than any single or combination of symptoms, warranting high priority for colonoscopic follow-up.

Majority of CRCs are endoluminal adenocarcinomas that arise from the mucosa. Colonoscopy is the most versatile diagnostic test in symptomatic individuals. Computed tomography (CT) colonography provides a similarly sensitive, less invasive alternative to colonoscopy in patients presenting with symptoms suggestive of CRC. However, given that colonoscopy permits removal/biopsy of the lesion and any synchronous cancers or polyps that are seen during the same procedure, colonoscopy remains the gold standard for investigation of symptoms suggestive of CRC.

Once the diagnosis is established, a metastatic workup is done to provide a framework for discussing therapy and prognosis. Preoperative clinical staging is done with physical examination and CT scan of the chest, abdomen and pelvis. Serum carcinoembryonic antigen (CEA) level is obtained preoperatively and postoperatively in patients with demonstrated CRC to aid treatment planning and assessment of prognosis.

Patients should have a colonoscopic examination of the entire colon prior to surgery. If full colonoscopy cannot be performed because of obstruction or poor preparation, the entire residual colon should be examined colonoscopically soon after resection. Surgical resection is the only curative modality for localized CRC. Endoscopic resection is a reasonable alternative to radical surgery for selected early stage CRC arising in a polyp, as long as they meet certain criteria for favorable risk. On recovery, adjuvant chemotherapy eradicates micrometastases, reduces the likelihood of disease recurrence, and increases cure rates. The benefits are clear with stage III (node-positive) CRC. In this setting, a six month course of oxaliplatin-based chemotherapy is generally recommended. The benefit of chemotherapy for resected stage II CRC is controversial, and treatment decisions must be individualized. Chemotherapy is associated with toxicities, including mucositis, emesis, diarrhea, febrile neutropenia, fatigue, hair loss, hand-foot syndrome, and cardiotoxicity. The frequency and severity of these side effects vary according to the specific drugs used and how they are administered, most are reversible when chemotherapy is discontinued. Most patients who present with metastatic disease are not surgical candidates, and palliative chemotherapy is generally recommended. However, surgery may provide a potentially curative option for selected patients with limited metastatic disease, predominantly in the liver and lung. An aggressive surgical approach to both the primary and the metastatic sites is warranted in such patients in conjunction with systemic chemotherapy. For patients with unresectable distant metastases, majority of patients without symptoms who initiate chemotherapy never require palliative surgery.

The most important indicator of outcome following resection of CRC is pathologic stage. After treatment for a stage II or III CRC, posttreatment surveillance consists of periodic history and physical examination and assay of the serum CEA, annual surveillance CT scans, and periodic colonoscopy. Following treatment for stage I CRC, posttreatment surveillance consists only of periodic history and physical examination and colonoscopy.

5. Lung Cancer

Lung cancer remains the most common cause of cancer mortality for both men and women worldwide. In 2018, it affected 2.1 million patients and caused 1.7 million deaths. The biggest risk factor is cigarette smoking; responsible for approximately 90 percent of cases of lung cancer (secondhand smoke is also a significant cause of lung cancer). Hence prevention and cessation of smoking offer the most important route to decreasing the morbidity and mortality associated with this disease. Numerous occupational and environmental carcinogens increase the risk of lung cancer, best known are asbestos and radon. In the developing world, additional risk factors, such as smoke and air pollution are important.

Lung cancer is the leading cause of cancer death in black men and women in North America. After increasing for decades, lung cancer death rates in black men began to decline in 1990, however rates in black women increased until the late 2000s but has decreased 1.1 percent annually over the past decade [14].

With increasing life expectancy in Africa, the burden of many cancers including lung cancer continues to increase. Unfortunately, cancer diagnosis rate in Africa remains low, with under-reporting, poor cancer registry information, and patients present usually in an advanced stage so the full magnitude of lung cancer is likely not captured [15]. Another study suggested lung cancer incidence rates are lower in Africa compared to incidence rates elsewhere, possibly due to a true lack of cases or detection biases [16].

Lung cancer is divided into non-small cell lung cancer (NSCLC) and small cell lung cancer (SCLC). NSCLC accounts for approximately 85 percent of lung cancers with the remainder being mostly SCLC.

The clinical manifestations of lung cancer are due to intrathoracic effects of the tumor such as cough, hemoptysis, pleural disease, extrathoracic metastases (liver, bone, brain), or paraneoplastic phenomena such as hypercalcemia, Cushing syndrome, hypercoagulability disorders and various neurologic syndromes.

Most patients present for diagnostic evaluation because of symptoms suspicious for lung cancer or an incidental finding on chest imaging. The goal of initial evaluation is to obtain sufficient clinical and radiologic information to guide diagnostic tissue biopsy, staging, and treatment.

Every patient with suspected lung cancer should undergo CT scan of the chest and upper abdomen (contrast-enhanced) to evaluate the extent of the primary tumor and potential spread to the mediastinum, liver, and adrenal glands. For NSCLC, where possible, PET or PET/CT is performed in patients who are resection candidates with larger primary lesions (T2 or T3 by CT scan), or in those at high risk for surgical complications as the use of PET may reduce the incidence of futile thoracotomies.

A diagnosis of lung cancer is made by pathologic evaluation of cytologic (pleural fluid) or tissue biopsy. Initial radiographic staging guides the selection of a biopsy site and preferred modality to obtain a pathologic sample. It is important to obtain a large enough sample to allow supplemental immunohistochemical and genetic analysis. Adenocarcinoma, squamous carcinoma, adenosquamous carcinoma, and large cell carcinoma are the four major histological subtypes of NSCLC.

For NSCLC patients with early stage disease, surgical resection offers the best opportunity for cure, while concurrent chemoradiotherapy is preferred with more extensive intrathoracic disease. Patients with advanced disease are managed palliatively with systemic therapy and/or local palliative modalities. SCLC is disseminated at presentation in almost all patients, hence systemic chemotherapy is important in all stages. With limited-stage disease, thoracic XRT is used in combination with chemotherapy. Prophylactic cranial XRT is recommended to decrease the incidence of brain metastases and prolong survival. Prophylactic cranial XRT and thoracic XRT is also beneficial in those with complete or partial response to initial systemic chemotherapy.

A minority of patients with NSCLC have pathologic stage I and II disease when diagnosed. Importantly, early-stage disease is curable with aggressive therapy. For patients with adequate pulmonary function and without serious medical comorbidity, surgical resection is the preferred initial treatment for patients with stage I or II NSCLC rather than XRT. Adjuvant chemotherapy with a platinum based doublet after complete resection of stage II NSCLC and stage IB NSCLC with high-risk features is standard.

Stage III NSCLC is a highly heterogeneous group of patients with differences in the extent and localization of disease. A multidisciplinary approach is essential for management of stage III disease. For one small subset of Stage III NSCLC (T3N1), surgery is indicated if complete resection is technically feasible, with adjuvant chemotherapy following resection. For patients with N2 disease, standard is to treat with concurrent chemoradiotherapy, using platinum-based chemotherapy (cisplatin/carboplatin with etoposide/paclitaxel) plus full-dose XRT. With N3 disease, concurrent chemoradiotherapy and consolidation durvalumab is the standard.

Lung cancer survivors are at risk for recurrence of their original cancer, the development of second primary lung cancers, and the development of other cancers, particularly those related to smoking. Close surveillance is required for survivors to detect such malignancies at an early stage. Smoking cessation is indicated both to decrease the risk of a second primary malignancy and to reduce comorbidity. Patients should receive cessation counseling, advice, and pharmacotherapy.

Advanced NSCLC requires sequential use of systemic therapies in an effort to prolong overall survival while maintaining quality of life. Available systemic therapy options include immunotherapy, cytotoxic chemotherapy, biologics, and targeted agents. Factors that influence the choice and sequence of therapies for an individual patient include histology (squamous versus non-squamous), the presence or absence of driver mutations, and performance status and preferences regarding treatment. Tumor tissue is assessed for expression of programmed cell death ligand 1 (PD-L1) expression. Patients with non-squamous NSCLC should also have their tumor tested for the presence of a driver mutation, such as mutated epidermal growth factor receptor (EGFR), the anaplastic lymphoma kinase (ALK) fusion oncogene, and other targetable mutations. If tumor contains a driver mutation, use of a specific inhibitor is recommended and if tolerated, continued until there is evidence of progressive disease. Immunotherapy-based approaches are not appropriate as first-line treatment for these patients.

Treatment for patients whose tumor does not contain a driver mutation depends on the level of expression of PD-L1. For most patients with advanced, non-squamous or squamous NSCLC, and high PD-L1 expression ($\geq$50 percent of tumor cells with staining), standard first-line treatment is with pembrolizumab or atezolizumab monotherapy. However, for those with rapidly progressive disease or high tumor burden, standard treatment is concurrent chemotherapy and immunotherapy. For tumors with low or intermediate PD-L1 expression (<50 percent of tumor cells with staining), the standard is histology-appropriate, platinum-based chemotherapy doublet with immunotherapy (shown to improve survival compared with chemotherapy alone). For non-squamous NSCLC, the combination of either cisplatin or carboplatin with pemetrexed is standard and for squamous NSCLC, a combination of carboplatin with paclitaxel or nabpaclitaxel and pembrolizumab is standard.

In addition to systemic therapy, treatment directed at specific sites of metastases and toward symptom control is important with overall patient management.

6. Cervical Cancer

In 2018, cervical cancer accounted for an estimated 570,000 new cancer cases and 311,000 deaths worldwide and was the fourth most common cancer in women. 84 percent of cervical cancer cases are from less developed regions. In countries that do not have access to cervical cancer screening and prevention programs, cervical cancer remains the second most common type of cancer and third most common cause of cancer deaths among all types of cancer in women.

In North America, an estimated 2250 cases of invasive cervical cancer were diagnosed in black women in 2019. The incidence of cervical cancer is 30 percent higher in black women than white women, however this racial disparity has narrowed over the past several decades. Black women are still more likely than white women to be diagnosed with more advanced disease hence 5 year survival among black women is 56 percent compared to 68 percent in their white counterparts [14].

Cervical cancer is the second most common cancer and the leading cause of cancer death in SSA women. A review of cervical cancer incidence over a period of 10 to 25 years from 10 population-based cancer registries across eight SSA countries reveals that cervical cancer incidence has been increasing in most of SSA [17].

Human papillomavirus (HPV) is central to the development of cervical neoplasia and can be detected in almost 100 percent of cervical cancers. Subtypes HPV 16 and 18 are found in over 70 percent of all cervical cancers. The most common histologic types of cervical cancer are squamous cell (70 percent) and adenocarcinoma (25 percent). Risk factors for cervical cancer are mostly associated with an increased risk of acquiring or having a compromised immune response to HPV infection; early onset of sexual activity, multiple sexual partners, a high-risk sexual partner, history of sexually transmitted infections, history of vulvar or vaginal squamous intraepithelial neoplasia or cancer, and immunosuppression. Oral contraceptive use appears to be associated with an increased risk of cervical cancer. Cigarette smoking appears to be associated with an increased risk of squamous cell cancer but not adenocarcinoma.

Early cervical cancer is frequently asymptomatic, emphasizing the importance of screening. The most common symptoms at presentation are abnormal vaginal bleeding (including postcoital bleeding) and vaginal discharge. A lesion may or may not be visible or palpable on physical examination. The diagnosis of cervical cancer is established by biopsy. Symptomatic patients without a visible lesion and those who have only abnormal cervical cytology should undergo colposcopy with directed biopsy and, if necessary, diagnostic conization.

Early-stage cervical cancer includes stages IA, IB1, and IB2 disease and is determined by the depth of stromal invasion and the overall tumor size. For women with microinvasive disease (stage IA1) treatment with conization or extrafascial hysterectomy rather than radical hysterectomy is adequate. For women of reproductive age who wish to preserve their fertility and have a lesion size $\leq$2 cm and no lymph node metastases, uterus-preserving surgery is reasonable. For women with stage IA2 and IB1 cervical cancer, modified radical hysterectomy is recommended. For stage IB2 disease radical hysterectomy is recommended. Lymph node assessment is performed for stages IA2 to IB2 disease. Primary XRT, with or without chemotherapy is used for women who are not candidates for primary surgery due to medical comorbidities or poor functional status. Laparotomy for radical hysterectomy has better oncologic outcomes than minimally invasive surgery for many women. For women with early-stage cervical cancer with intermediate-risk features (lymphovascular invasion, cervical stromal invasion, or tumor size ≥4 cm), adjuvant chemoradiation rather than XRT alone is used.

For women with early-stage cervical cancer with high-risk features (positive surgical margins, pathologically involved pelvic nodes, or positive involvement of the parametria), adjuvant chemoradiation is used. Adjuvant XRT is given with single-agent cisplatin rather than the combination of cisplatin plus fluorouracil.

Locally advanced cervical cancer includes disease confined to the cervix with a clinically visible tumor >4 cm (stage IB3); disease that invades beyond the uterus, but involves less than the upper two-thirds of the vagina (stage II); disease that extends to the pelvic sidewall, involves the lower third of vagina, and/or causes hydronephrosis or nonfunctioning kidney (stage III); or disease that extends to the rectum or bladder, or beyond the true pelvis (stage IVA). Primary chemoradiation is preferred but primary surgery, neoadjuvant chemotherapy followed by surgery, or radiation therapy are also reasonable treatment options. Ideally a PET or CT is performed in all patients with locally advanced cervical cancer in order to better define the extent of disease and evaluate the pelvic and para-aortic lymph nodes.

For women with recurrent cervical cancer that are not surgical candidates, and women who present initially with metastatic disease, first-line treatment with platinum-based combination chemotherapy (usually cisplatin plus paclitaxel) is recommended. Carboplatin plus paclitaxel is a good alternative, for patients who are poor candidates for cisplatin and patients previously treated with cisplatin-based chemoradiation.

Cervical cancer is highly preventable and PAP testing picks up cervical abnormalities in preinvasive rather than invasive cancer stage. Worldwide, cervical cancer is the fourth most common cancer of women with case numbers declining in regions where screening programs have been implemented. Vaccines have been developed to protect against acquisition of HPV infection and development of subsequent HPV-associated disease such as cervical cancer. However, in resource-poor areas, where screening programs and HPV vaccines are not well established, cervical cancer continues to affect and kill hundreds of thousands of women.

7. Hepatocellular Cancer (HCC)

Cancer of the liver and intrahepatic bile ducts is the sixth common cancer worldwide, with approximately 841,000 new cases reported in 2018. HCC is the fourth leading cause of cancer-related mortality worldwide, with over 780,000 deaths in 2018. HCC is more common in men (male to female ratio 3:1). Patients with cirrhosis from any etiology are at risk for developing HCC and up to one-third of patients with cirrhosis will develop HCC during their lifetime. Nonalcoholic fatty liver disease (NAFLD) and nonalcoholic steatohepatitis (NASH) related cirrhosis, are risk factors for HCC in Western countries. Vaccination against hepatitis B virus (HBV) infection can prevent infection, and protects against HBV-related HCC. Patients with chronic HBV or HCV infection who are successfully treated with antiviral therapy have reduced HCC risk.

There are race-related and ethnicity-related differences in HCC incidence, surveillance, diagnosis, and treatment in the United States. African Americans have an elevated incidence of HCC and high HCC-related mortality. Between 2005 and 2007, HCC incidence rates in African Americans was more than 1.5 times higher than the national average. Also, African Americans have lower rates of HCC screening than patients of other races, present with more advanced HCC and are offered curative surgical therapy less often than members of other races. African American patients have significantly higher in-hospital HCC-related mortality than whites, as well as decreased overall survival [18].

HCC is the fourth most common cancer on the African continent, where there are differences between North Africa and SSA. HCC incidence in Egypt is two-fold higher than in SSA, due to the unusually high prevalence in Egypt (4.6 percent in men) of HCV infection. Hepatitis B and C are the most important risk factors for HCC in Africa. Aflatoxin has been shown to be important either as a stand-alone risk factor or in synergism with HBV and HCV infection in the initiation of HCC. Given the increasing adoption of a western lifestyle in Africa with an associated increase in obesity and type 2 diabetes mellitus, the contribution of NAFLD/NASH as a risk factor for HCC is expected to rise. The 2016 global health strategy of the World Health Organization (WHO) on viral hepatitis aims to achieve a 90 percent reduction in new cases of chronic hepatitis B and C, and to reduce mortality due to hepatitis B and C by 65 percent by 2030. Viral hepatitis accounts for over 80 percent of all liver cancers in Africa [19].

There is a range of clinical presentations for patients with HCC, from being asymptomatic to presenting with a life-threatening illness such as variceal hemorrhage. Previously stable patients with cirrhosis may develop features of decompensation (variceal bleeding or ascites) due to the extension of HCC into the hepatic or portal veins. Patients with HCC can develop a paraneoplastic syndrome that can manifest as hypoglycemia, erythrocytosis, hypercalcemia and diarrhea. HCC can be diagnosed on contrast-enhanced CT, MRI, or ultrasound. In high-risk patients, HCC can sometimes be diagnosed with imaging alone. In a non-high-risk patient, a liver lesion usually requires further evaluation (serum tumor markers and biopsy) for definitive diagnosis. Following HCC diagnosis, review preferably in a multidisciplinary setting, is ideal to decide on therapy.

The preferred therapy for localized HCC is surgical resection, but majority of patients are not eligible because of tumor extent or underlying liver dysfunction. For patients who are not surgically resectable, liver transplantation is the only other potentially curative option. Unfortunately most patients who are considered for liver transplantation are unresectable because of the degree of underlying liver dysfunction rather than tumor extent. For patients with liver-isolated disease who are not eligible for resection or transplantation, treatment options include local nonsurgical methods of liver-directed tumor thermal ablation, embolization, percutaneous injection therapy, external beam radiation therapy, and systemic therapy. The selection of treatment option is determined by the severity of underlying liver disease, the size and distribution of the intrahepatic tumors, the vascular supply, and the patient's overall performance status and also availability. Locoregional forms of therapy are preferable to systemic therapy for initial treatment of patients with locally advanced unresectable HCC. In patients who progress after locoregional therapy, additional liver-directed therapy may be possible depending on tumor location and underlying liver function. Once locoregional therapy is exhausted, systemic therapy is the only option if performance status and underlying liver function are adequate.

Until 2008, there was no effective therapy for patients with advanced HCC or those failing local therapies. There is now data showing that molecularly targeted agents sorafenib and regorafenib improve survival versus best supportive care alone. Subsequently, a survival benefit has also been shown in the second-line setting with nivolumab (immune checkpoint inhibitor); lenvatinib has demonstrated noninferiority to first-line sorafenib, and the combination of atezolizumab plus bevacizumab has demonstrated superiority to first-line sorafenib. These results have changed the treatment landscape for advanced HCC. Second-line therapy is an option for patients whose tumors progress while receiving a molecularly targeted agent and whose performance status and liver function are sufficient to tolerate it. Supportive care alone is appropriate for those with poor liver function or extensive comorbidity.

8. Sickle Cell Disease (SCD)

SCD is an inherited group of disorders uniquely present in blacks and characterized by the presence of hemoglobin S (HbS), either from homozygosity for the sickle mutation in the beta globin chain of hemoglobin (HbSS) or from compound heterozygosity of a sickle beta globin mutation with another beta globin mutation (e.g., sickle-beta thalassemia). Diagnosis of one of the sickle cell disorders is made via high performance liquid chromatography (HPLC), isoelectric focusing (IEF), or gel electrophoresis techniques. In prenatal diagnosis and in areas with high frequency of non-sickle-cell disorders, polymerase chain reaction (PCR) techniques, or direct DNA testing may be used. The hallmarks of SCD are vaso-occlusive phenomena and hemolytic anemia and many other complications that can be life threatening. Sickle cell trait is a benign carrier condition characterized by heterozygosity for the sickle hemoglobin mutation.

SCD carries orphan disease designation in the United States, with about 2000 affected infants born annually and fewer than 100,000 persons living with this condition. More than 75 percent of the global burden of SCA occurs in SSA, where scarce health resources and inadequate awareness among health care providers and the general public contribute to high rates of early mortality [20]. SCD is a common and growing health problem in many parts of SSA, where at least 240,000 affected children are born with the condition every year. Here, SCD is widely neglected and an estimated 50 percent to 90 percent of those born with the condition die undiagnosed before their fifth birthdays. A likely large proportion of these deaths are attributable to 2 main conditions: malaria and invasive bacterial infections. A greater emphasis on basic and applied research in the area of SCD in SSA would lead to life improvements to the many affected people and their families [21].

Patients with SCD should be seen regularly by a clinician and treatment team as part of a comprehensive health care maintenance program. Hydroxyurea is the mainstay of treatment for SCD, it reduces pain and other vaso-occlusive complications, decreases hospitalization rates, and improves survival. Other options including glutamine, voxelotor, and crizanlizumab are available for patients who cannot tolerate hydroxyurea or who have continued pain despite hydroxyurea. Hematopoietic cell transplantation (HCT) is the only available curative option in individuals with SCD. Indications for blood transfusion are preparation for surgery; treatment of symptomatic anemia, acute stroke, multiorgan failure, acute chest syndrome; prevention of stroke and acute chest syndrome and recurrent priapism. All patients with SCD should receive age appropriate vaccinations, including Streptococcus pneumoniae, seasonal influenza, Neisseria meningitidis, Haemophilus influenzae type B, and hepatitis B.

Supplementation with folic acid, multivitamin (without iron), vitamin D and calcium, which are often deficient is suggested.

While survival with SCD is reduced compared with the general population, the prognosis for SCD has been improving following the institution of comprehensive care: Where available, the disease has shifted from a fatal pediatric illness to a chronic disease often associated with progressive deterioration in quality-of-life and organ function. Survival well into adulthood for those with access to comprehensive care is well documented. In a 2014 cohort study of African Americans at a tertiary care medical center, the median survival for HbSS and HbSβ0 was 58 years, and median survival for HbSC and HbSβ+ was 66 years [22]. In a recent British study of over 700 adults, the median survival for HbSS and HbSβ0 was 67 years [23]. This improved survival was attributed to care at a specialist hematology clinic, inpatient management by a dedicated team, involvement of specialists in other organ systems, availability of on-site red blood cell (RBC) exchange, and a focused "transition program" to facilitate safe transition from pediatric to adult care. Generally, the median life span of SCD patients in the United States is about 43 years with a similar trend towards improved survival [24]. Patients who survive into later adulthood can have long-term disease complications not seen in younger patients including renal insufficiency which may occur in 85 percent of individuals.

9. Areas for Improvement in Cancer Care of Older African Adults

In 2017, twenty-one percent of African-Americans compared to nine percent of Caucasians were living below the poverty line in the United States. Because of historical context and social structure, race is strongly correlated with socioeconomic status in the United States and, socioeconomic status is the most critical factor affecting health and longevity. Socioeconomic status influences cancer care and outcomes across the cancer continuum from prevention to palliative care. Unfortunately, socioeconomic disparities in cancer mortality have widened over the past several decades for all cancers combined: Access to healthcare influences the use of preventative and early detection services as well as receiving cancer treatment and survivor care. In United States, healthcare access is closely related to insurance coverage and without coverage or poor coverage, all cancer care outcomes are worse. Compared to Caucasians, African-Americans are more likely to be uninsured and less likely to have private insurance [14].

In SSA, advances with the prevention and treatment of malaria and HIV have helped people live longer; cancer rates are now on the rise given longer lifespan in SSA. Most of SSA which consists of 48 countries south of the Sahara desert have limited medical resources; for example, many hospitals in this region have limited access to cancer surgeons, radiation therapy machines and drug treatments including painkillers. Hence cancers are often not diagnosed until they are more advanced. Several agencies have developed cancer care guidelines for SSA that try to take into account the context in which care is being provided [25].

A good example is the WHO which launched the 2013 global action plan for prevention and control of non-communicable diseases; that aims to reduce a quarter of premature mortality from cancer (along with other non-communicable illnesses) by 2025. This is to be achieved by increasing political commitment for cancer prevention and control, coordinating and conducting research on the causes of human cancer and mechanisms of carcinogenesis, monitoring the cancer burden, identifying priority stages for cancer prevention and control, generating new knowledge and disseminate existing knowledge to facilitate delivery of evidence-based approaches to cancer care, developing standards and tools to guide the planning and implementation of interventions for prevention, early diagnosis, screening, treatment, palliative care and survivorship. Facilitating broad networks of cancer control partners and experts at global, regional and national levels, strengthening health systems at national and local levels to deliver cure and care for cancer patients, providing global leadership as well as technical assistance to support governments and their partners build and sustain high quality cancer control programs; and providing technical assistance for rapid, effective transfer of best practice interventions to less developed countries [26]. This is a commendable albeit ambitious plan and is a good start for developing countries including those in SSA.

For patients with an advanced, serious and/or life-threatening illness such as cancer, palliative care is an interdisciplinary collaboration that focuses on patient defined goals of care and relief of the patients' and families' distress. While palliative care used to be seen as care that was provided for people who were not receiving any active treatment for advanced illness, and were in fact dying of their disease, the principles of palliative care are equally applicable to early stage, potentially curable disease and should be provided alongside disease modifying treatment.

For the overwhelming majority of Africans who currently endure life-limiting illnesses such as terminal cancer, access to culturally appropriate holistic palliative care (including effective pain management) is not available. A survey of hospice and palliative care services on the continent found that 45 percent of African countries had no identified hospice or palliative care activity, and only 9 percent could be classified as having services approaching some measure of integration with mainstream health provision. This vast unmet need for palliative care can only be addressed by the public health approach to palliative care delivery advocated by the WHO and supported by African palliative care association [27].

References

[1] The Burden of Cancer | The Cancer Atlas https://canceratlas.cancer.org/the-burden/the-burden-of-cancer. *American Cancer Society*, Inc. 2019.

[2] Bollyky TJ. *The Growing Cancer Threat in Africa*. https://www.thinkglobalhealth.org/article/growing-cancer-threat-africa. February 4, 2020.

[3] Sub-Saharan Africa | The Cancer Atlas https://canceratlas.cancer.org/the-burden/sub-saharan-africa. *American Cancer Society*, Inc. 2019.

[4] Parkin DM, Bray F, Ferlay J, Jemal A. Cancer in Africa 2012. *Cancer Epidemiol Biomarkers Prev*. 2014 Jun; 23(6):953-66.

[5] DeSantis CE, Miller KD, Goding Sauer A, Jemal A, Siegel RL. Cancer statistics for African Americans, 2019. *CA Cancer J Clin.* 2019 May; 69(3):211-233.

[6] Kesson EM, Allardice GM, George WD, Burns HJ, Morrison DS. Effects of multidisciplinary team working on breast cancer survival: retrospective, comparative, interventional cohort study of 13 722 women. *BMJ*. 2012 Apr 26; 344:e2718.

[7] *Breast Cancer Rates among Black Women and White Women*. https://www.cdc.gov/cancer/dcpc/research/articles/breast_cancer_rates_women.htm. Oct 13, 2016 (Last reviewed Nov 2020).

[8] Adeloye D, Sowunmi OY, Jacobs W et al. Estimating the incidence of breast cancer in Africa: a systematic review and meta-analysis. *J Glob Health*. 2018 Jun; 8(1):010419.

[9] Caswell-Jin JL, Plevritis SK, Tian L, Cadham CJ, Xu C, Stout NK, Sledge GW, Mandelblatt JS, Kurian AW. Change in Survival in Metastatic Breast Cancer with Treatment Advances: Meta-Analysis and Systematic Review. *JNCI Cancer Spectr*. 2018 Nov; 2(4):pky062.

[10] Jim Stallard. *4 Things African American Men Should Know about Prostate Cancer.* April 23, 2019. https://www.mskcc.org/news/4-things-african-american-men-should-know-about-prostate.

[11] Adeloye D, David RA, Aderemi AV et al. An Estimate of the Incidence of Prostate Cancer in Africa: A Systematic Review and Meta-Analysis. *PLoS One*. 2016 Apr 13; 11(4):e0153496.

[12] Augustus GJ, Ellis NA. Colorectal Cancer Disparity in African Americans Risk Factors and Carcinogenic Mechanisms. *Am J Pathol.* 2018 Feb; 188(2):291-303.

[13] Graham A, Adeloye D, Grant L, Theodoratou E, Campbell H. Estimating the incidence of colorectal cancer in Sub–Saharan Africa: A systematic analysis. *J Glob Health*. 2012 Dec; 2(2):020404.

[14] *Cancer Facts & Figures for African Americans 2019-2021.* https://www.cancer.org/content/dam/cancer-org/research/cancer-facts-and-statistics/cancer-facts-and-figures-for-african-americans/cancer-facts-and-figures-for-african-americans-2019-2021.pdf. American Cancer Society, Inc. 2019.

[15] Gaafar R. Lung Cancer in Africa: Challenges and Perspectives. *J Thorac Oncol.* 2017 Jan 01, Volume 12, Issue 1, Supplement, S115-S116.

[16] Urman A, Josyula S, Rosenberg A, Lounsbury D, Rohan T, Hosgood HD. Burden of Lung Cancer and Associated Risk Factors in Africa by Region., *J Pulm Respir Med* 2016, Volume 6: Issue 3.

[17] Jedy-Agba E, Joko WY, Liu B et al. Trends in cervical cancer incidence in sub-Saharan Africa. *Br J Cancer.* 2020 Jul; 123(1):148-154.

[18] Winters AC, Sung JC, Wyatt B et al. At Diagnosis of Hepatocellular Carcinoma, African Americans With Hepatitis C Have Better Liver Function Than Other Patients. *Clin Liver Dis* (Hoboken). 2018 Oct; 12(4):109-112.

[19] Okeke E, Davwar PM, Roberts L et al. Epidemiology of Liver Cancer in Africa: Current and Future Trends. *Semin Liver Dis.* 2020 May; 40(2):111-123.

[20] McGann PT, Hernandez AG, Ware RE. Sickle cell anemia in sub-Saharan Africa: advancing the clinical paradigm through partnerships and research. *Blood.* 2017 Jan 12; 129(2):155-161.

[21] Williams TN. Sickle Cell Disease in Sub-Saharan Africa. *Hematol Oncol Clin North Am.* 2016 Apr; 30(2):343-58.

[22] Elmariah H, Garrett ME, De Castro LM et al. Factors associated with survival in a contemporary adult sickle cell disease cohort. *Am J Hematol.* 2014 May; 89(5):530-5.

[23] Gardner K, Douiri A, Drasar E et al. Survival in adults with sickle cell disease in a high-income setting. *Blood.* 2016 Sep 8; 128(10):1436-8.

[24] Payne AB, Mehal JM, Chapman C et al. Trends in Sickle Cell Disease-Related Mortality in the United States, 1979 to 2017. *Ann Emerg Med.* 2020 Sep; 76(3S):S28-S36.

[25] Walker C. *Improving Cancer Care in Sub-Saharan Africa*. https://www.cancertodaymag.org/Pages/Spring2018/Improving-Cancer-Care-in-Sub-Saharan-Africa.aspx. March 22, 2018.

[26] Cancer. https://www.afro.who.int/health-topics/cancer. *World Health Organization* 2020.

[27] African Palliative Care Association. *Palliative care in Africa: the need.* https://www.africanpalliativecare.org/awareness/palliative-care-in-africa-the-need/ 2020.

In: Care of the Older African Adult
Editor: Seki A. Balogun
ISBN: 978-1-53619-295-7

Chapter 7

NEUROPSYCHIATRIC DISORDERS IN OLDER BLACK ADULTS

Mudhasir Bashir*
Associate Professor
Department of Psychiatry and Neurobehavioral Sciences
University of Virginia Health System
Charlottesville, VA, US

ABSTRACT

Neuropsychiatric disorders are a major public health problem and a leading cause of disability worldwide. They impose a high personal and social cost, in addition to contributing significantly to the global burden of disease. We face an ageing world population, a large subgroup of which is the black population. This group has a high burden of risk factors including chronic illnesses, lower education and other structural social factors. They face increased socioeconomic disadvantage, everyday discrimination and other disparities that affect quality of life and predispose them to psychiatric disorders. There is also a tremendous paucity of systematic data on the identification, recognition, treatment and management of mental

* Corresponding Author's Email: MB5QD@hscmail.mcc.virginia.edu.

disorders in this population. Research for mental disorders in older black adults is particularly limited. Tremendous disparities exist for the older black adult in being able to access and use mental health services. Major public health policy efforts are needed to address these issues. This chapter will try to address some of the challenges to be cognizant of in the treatment of neuropsychiatric disorders in the older black population.

Keywords: mental disorders, psychiatric illness, geriatric, older adults, African American, Black, depression, mood disorders, dementias, anxiety, schizophrenia spectrum disorders, psychosis, epidemiologic studies, prevalence, screening.

1. EPIDEMIOLOGY

According to the US Census Bureau report from September 2020, the older black population is projected to triple from 74.4 million to 235.1 million by 2050. The older non-Hispanic African American population (age 65 and over) was 4,587,094 in 2017, and is projected to grow to 12.1 million by 2060. This bump will move Black Americans from 9% of the older population to 13% in the next three decades.

Caring for this growing older black population will mean understanding their unmet needs in both mental and physical health, which are closely intertwined. The challenges that come with psychiatric disorders are not only personal but also financial, social, and familial. This is particularly true of those in the lower socioeconomic strata where the older black population are at greatest risk. Per the United States Census Bureau, the poverty rate in 2016 for African Americans age 65 and older was 18.7%, double the rate of 9.3% for all older Americans. Other risk factors in this population include lower education levels, racial bias and societal discrimination.

Addressing issues of mental health in older Blacks is made more difficult by the fact that there are very few large scale studies that specifically involve this demographic. The Collaborative Psychiatric Epidemiologic Survey (CPES) that links three data sets - the National Comorbidity Survey-Replication (NCS-R), the National Latino and Asian

American Study (NLAAS) and the National Survey of American Life (NSAL) addressed some of these issues. The NSAL was designed to be representative of Blacks in the United States. Although still small in numbers and now fifteen years old, the CPES has provided information of prevalence and other correlates of psychiatric disorders in African Americans [1]. Using data from the NSAL, Ford et al. indicated that 23% of older African Americans reported at least one lifetime psychiatric disorder and 8.54% reported at least one disorder over 12 months. The most prevalent disorders over 12 months in this subgroup were Major Depressive Disorder (MDD), Post-Traumatic Stress Disorder (PTSD) and social phobia [2]. A large study [3] showed that among African Americans with MDD, 44.9% had a lifetime anxiety disorder, 29.6% had lifetime dysthymia, 27.4% has a lifetime substance use disorder, and 25.5% reported lifetime suicidal ideation.

There is little data on suicide and suicidal behaviors in African Americans. Older African Americans with multiple psychiatric disorders are at greatest risk of suicide.[4] Chatters et al. using the NSAL data, estimated lifetime prevalence of suicidal ideation and attempts among older African Americans and black Caribbeans was 6.1% and 2.1%. One in four attempters and two in five ideators never had treatment for mental health.

Inadequate treatment of psychiatric issues in the older black population is the result of a number of factors including poor recognition, using invalid criteria, inadequate screening language, racial and nonracial discrimination, limited resources, poor utilization, and limited data on how to best treat this population. Most treatments use data extrapolated from studies that do not accurately represent the black population.

The population of older African Americans and blacks worldwide will continue to grow over the next few decades, and with it the prevalent comorbid psychiatric disorders. Research efforts towards this demographic needs to be more robust if we are to meet the challenges of the future in the care of older black adults.

2. Screening for Psychiatric Illnesses

Older adults tend to present to their primary care providers for health concerns. These visits are the opportunity to screen them for the most common mental health symptoms including depression, anxiety, memory loss, psychotic symptoms, and functional decline. Many screening tools, such as the Geriatric Depression Scale (GDS) and Patient-Reported Outcomes Measurement Information System (PROMIS Global-10), are helpful in this population but should be interpreted with caution in the black population, as some language may not be consistent with cultural sensitivities. The Diagnostic and Statistical Manual of Mental Disorders (DSM) is used most widely to diagnose mental illness, but the language has been found to be inadequate in capturing symptoms of depression amongst African American older adults [5]. Given the prevalence of psychiatric disorders, the threshold for diagnosis should be low and consultation with a psychiatrist may prove to be valuable when in doubt.

3. Common Psychiatric Disorders

3.1. Mood Disorders

At the end of the next decade, depression is projected to become the leading cause of disability and second leading contributor to the global burden of disease. Depression in late life has a high association with suffering, disability, suicide risk, decreased health related quality of life, morbidity, and mortality. In the United States, a large study by Woodward et al. 2013 [3], showed that among African Americans with Major Depressive Disorder, 29.6% had lifetime dysthymia. Another study in rural South Africa showed that older age was the strongest correlate of depressive symptoms in those age 80 and older, indicating a particularly high need for depression screening and treatment among older adults in rural South Africa [6]. Subsyndromal depression may be more common in late life than major depression. Bipolar depression has the same prevalence across the lifespan.

The clinical presentation of late-life depression in African Americans is highly variable. African Americans tend to report less dysphoria[7], but more hopelessness and somatic symptoms than whites [8]. African Americans may conceptualize depression in a different manner, have different health beliefs about depression, or attach greater stigma to mental illness, all of which affect responses on self-rated depression scales [9]. These variations in the clinical presentation of depression underscore the need for using precise measurement instruments within this demographic.

Black older adults are at higher risk for misdiagnosis, under-treatment, and more severe symptomatology than other groups [10]. Depressed older African Americans perceive their physical health more negatively and also tend to take less care of their general health. A study in South Africa showed a high risk of malnutrition is associated with depressive symptoms [11]. Comorbidity between psychiatric disorders and physical health problems is high. Studies suggest that African American women in particular tend to believe depression to be a normal reaction to life circumstances and do not seek professional help. They instead cope by use of culturally sanctioned behavior including religious practices and resilience [12]. In another study, African American men had difficulty distinguishing between stress and depression [13]. African Americans are also more likely to anticipate stigma for mental disorders and view depression as part of the normal aging process [14]. Barriers to identification and treatment of depression include poor access to quality mental health, stigma of mental illness, mistrust of mental health providers and poor provider client communication

Approach to treatment of depression for older Blacks is no different than their white peers. It starts with accurate screening using valid screening tools. The Geriatric Depression Scale (GDS) is widely used for screening of depression in older adults in general, with the caveats of language insensitivities mentioned above. The GDS-SF (short form) has been shown to be more reliable [15]. Other studies have supported the internal validity and test-retest reliability of this screen in African American older adults as well [16]. The Center for Epidemiological Studies Depression scale (CES-D) has also shown validity in older adults. A group-specific three-item brief CES-D score has emerged as a reliable measure in Puerto Ricans and

African American older adults in some studies [17]. The PHQ-2 is a valid screening tool for major depression in older adults but should be followed by a more comprehensive diagnostic process. Specificity differences due to race appear to be insignificant [18].

Antidepressant medications form the mainstay of depression management. Selective Serotonin Reuptake Inhibitors (SSRIs) have largely replaced tricyclic antidepressants (TCAs) and Monoamine Oxidase Inhibitors (MAOIs), and are widely used as antidepressants of choice due to their good safety profile and lower rate of medication interactions. TCAs and MAOIs are used in rare cases, but require a high degree of vigilance as they have significant side effects and interactions. MAOIs also necessitate dietary restrictions. Unfortunately, African Americans are less likely to be prescribed antidepressants than their Caucasian peers despite the fact that SSRIs and SNRIs (Serotonin Norepinephrine Reuptake Inhibitors) are equally effective in the older Blacks as in Caucasians. Nonadherence, for which the most common issues are tolerability and cost, should be addressed at every visit. Augmentations to antidepressants, including mood stabilizers and other modalities, should be used judiciously but without reservation while making sure there are no interactions with other medications. The American Geriatrics Society Beers criteria is an invaluable guide to follow, to avoid using potentially inappropriate medications in older adults. Clinicians must be cognizant of dose titration in patients with liver or renal disease. A golden rule to always follow when prescribing for older adults is start low and go slow. If medication treatments are not effective after optimizing dosage, electroconvulsive therapy (ECT) and transcranial magnetic stimulation (TMS) are very effective tools to consider. They are generally underused in older adults and there is a higher disparity for black people, as depressed black inpatients continue to be far less likely than whites to receive ECT [19]. Therapy is less likely to be prescribed and less likely to be used by the African American population but has shown equal effectiveness [20].

The goal of treatment should be full recovery from depression and not just remission of symptoms. Incomplete recovery often leads to relapse. Length of maintenance therapy should be carefully considered and discussed with patients as it is very likely they will stop treatment as soon as they start feeling better, which can lead to relapse. Educating family members must also be prioritized, as low perceived social support from family members and significant others correlates directly with depression[21]. Late life depression is a public health problem and untreated depression contributes to poor health outcomes and increased mortality. Attention should also be paid to the nutritional status of the patient, as a study in South Africa showed a high risk of malnutrition is associated with depressive symptoms [11]. Malnutrition can be a cause or consequence of depression and should be remedied since overall functioning of the patient is essential to full recovery.

3.2. Anxiety Disorders

Anxiety is highly prevalent in the older population and can cause substantial impairment in functioning. Despite this, less than 25% undergo treatment, particularly in the case of the African American population [22]. There is a high prevalence of anxiety in late life which is significantly associated with increased risk of death in persons aged 75 and older [23]. Studies show primary care physicians are less likely to identify older black Americans as anxious compared to white patients. An understanding of the role of ethnicity in the identification of anxiety is important for the screening and management of anxiety in older persons [24]. African Americans were 3.43 and 4.8 times more likely to have clinically significant depression and anxiety than Caucasians [25].

Anxiety is clinically defined as a disproportional fear or worry of a situation or problem. Common symptoms include mental symptoms of excessive fear, avoiding social situations, poor sleep, muscular tension, feeling weak, and preoccupations, along with physical symptoms of racing heart, difficulty breathing, shaking, perspiration, and gastrointestinal disturbance.

The most common forms of anxiety in older adults are generalized anxiety and simple phobias. In a study of predominantly black participants, 8.9% of the sample met criteria for a current phobia and 10.2% met criteria at some time in their life [26]. The prevalence rate for specific phobias range from 5.9% to 13.1% in older adults. The association of depression and anxiety is well recognized and tend to be highly comorbid. This combination results in greater symptom severity and more difficult response to treatment. Presence of one therefore requires careful screening for the other.

Anxiety disorders are also highly comorbid with alcohol use, benzodiazepine abuse, chronic pain, and insomnia. People with insomnia in particular, have greater depression and anxiety and poorer treatment outcomes. These cause significant impairment in functioning and wellbeing.

Anxiety scales such as the Brief Panic Disorder Scale have shown greater reliability and validity in Caucasians compared to African Americans. As with depression, cultural differences with language and expressions associated with anxiety disorders contribute to the difficulty of accurate diagnosis in primary care populations [27].

Anxiety disorders are primarily treated with SSRIs. Patients presenting to their primary care physicians are sometimes initially treated with benzodiazepines, which might bring quick and short term relief but lead to long-term problems including falls and effects on cognition. Older adults are also good candidates for various adjuvant therapies such as Cognitive Behavior Therapy (CBT). These treatments have a better remission rate when treated with a combination of SSRIs and various talk therapies. CBT has shown the best results for treatment of anxiety. Also notable is the Calmer Life Project, a partnership established between researchers and faith based and social service organizations, which uses CBT and incorporated religious/spiritual components for late life anxiety treatment [28].

Barriers to treatment in African Americans include cost of treatment, stigma, fears of therapy, mistrust of the medical system, feeling no need for treatment, and scheduling issues.

3.3. Psychotic Disorders

By definition, psychosis is the inability to distinguish reality from fantasy and includes hallucinations, delusions, and formal thought disorder.

The most common disorders that cause psychosis in older adults include delirium, dementia, mood disorders, and primary thought disorders [29].

The prevalence of psychotic symptoms in Africans is not clearly estimated. In 2013, a study in Kenya found the prevalence of one or more psychotic symptoms to be 13.9%, and two or more symptoms to be 3.8%. A 2004 study showed prevalence to be at 8% and 0.6%, respectively. A British study showed people from black ethnic minorities had an excess prevalence rate of psychosis compared with the white majority population [30].

Studies have shown variations in the reporting of psychosis by different ethnicities. African Americans are less likely to endorse visual hallucinations but endorsed auditory hallucinations more. Findings from the NLAAS and NSAL study that used the World Health Organization Composite International Diagnostic Interview psychotic symptom screener (WMH-CIDI) suggest that variations exist by race/ethnicity in both psychotic-like symptom endorsement and in self-reported attributions, as well as understanding for these symptoms on a psychosis screening instrument. Ethnic/racial differences could result from culturally sanctioned beliefs and idioms of distress, which deserve more attention in conducting culturally informed and responsive screening, assessment, and treatment [31].

Psychosis is one of the most common conditions in later life, with a lifetime risk of 23%. Despite its high prevalence, late-onset psychosis remains a diagnostic and treatment enigma. There are no reliable pathognomonic signs to distinguish primary or secondary psychosis. Primary psychosis is a diagnosis of exclusion and the clinician must rule out secondary causes. Approximately 60% of older patients with new incident psychosis have secondary psychosis. Treatment is geared towards the specific cause of psychosis and tailored based on comorbid conditions. Frequently, environmental and psychosocial interventions are first-line treatments with the judicious use of pharmacotherapy as needed [32].

The consensus statement on late-onset schizophrenia (illness onset after 40 years of age) and very-late-onset, schizophrenia-like psychosis (onset after 60 years) has been determined by the International Late Onset Schizophrenia Group. This group of patients are more likely to be women with better occupational and marital histories. They are more likely to have paranoid delusions and hallucinations, and less likely to have disorganization and negative symptoms [33]. Late-onset patients are more likely than their earlier-onset counterparts to complain of visual, tactile, and olfactory hallucinations; persecutory delusions; and third-person, running commentary, and accusatory or abusive auditory hallucinations [33]. In open studies, 48-61% of patients show full remission of psychotic symptoms with treatment, although poor compliance may render treatment in the community less successful [33]. Antipsychotic drugs (first generation and second generation) are a mainstay of therapy. Drug treatment should be started at very low doses and increases in dose should be made slowly. Typical late-onset patients will respond to dose amounts that are about one-quarter to one-half those given to early-onset patients. Very-late-onset cases may respond to dose amounts as low as one-tenth of those used in young adults. Use of depot medication at very low doses may be successful in ensuring compliance. With the exception of clozapine, whose use is problematic in older patients, the atypical antipsychotic agents are clearly advantageous in the treatment of late-onset patients because of the reduced likelihood of extrapyramidal symptoms and tardive dyskinesia for which older patients are at higher risk [33].

Psychosis is often accompanied by multiple medical issues which adds to the difficulty of treatment. A multidisciplinary collaborative approach is required which considers the psychosis, side effects of the medications, their interaction with other drugs, comorbid illnesses and metabolic side effects. Psychosocial interventions are also needed as much as medications.

Psychosis is one of the most common neuropsychiatric symptoms of dementia. Delusions can cause severe distress, as these are fixed beliefs that often revolve around beliefs of being in danger, infidelity by spouses, impostors replacing family members in their homes, poisoned food, or family members leaving them or being in danger. In Lewy body dementia, illusions in many different forms may be present. The patient may feel that there is someone sitting just outside of their visual field, but when they turn in that direction, there is no one there. There may also be a feeling that strangers live in one's house without permission [34].

Another frequent cause of dementia related psychosis in older adults is from Parkinson's disease (PD). Psychosis is one of the most disabling complications associated with PD, occurring in up to 30% of PD patients treated chronically with antiparkinsonian drugs. Visual hallucinations, with or without delirium and paranoid delusions, are the most frequent symptoms [35]. Behavioral symptoms such as anxiety, depression and psychosis are common in PD, and dementia occurs in about 90% of patients with PD [36].

Antipsychotics are the mainstay of treatment for psychosis of any etiology. Although there is a dearth of studies focusing on the response rate to antipsychotics in older black patients, general use suggests antipsychotics both first and second generation are equally effective. One study of Ziprasidone showed similar efficacy and safety in black patients with schizophrenia compared to white patients and overall populations [37]. All antipsychotics, and especially second generation antipsychotics, have a black box warning for use in older adults due to associated increased risk of cardiovascular events and death. As such, they should be used with utmost care. A new medication by the name of Pimavanserin, an atypical antipsychotic with a different mechanism of action, has also been approved for the treatment of psychosis in Parkinson's disease. It is particularly useful in PD as it does not significantly affect the dopaminergic receptors which has limited the use of other antipsychotics in PD.

Patients on long term antipsychotic treatments should be regularly monitored for metabolic syndrome and tardive dyskinesia. There should also be frequent reassessment of the need for continuing antipsychotics or regulating dosages. A golden rule is to prescribe the smallest possible dose for the shortest possible time. People living with schizophrenia in sub-Saharan Africa are often treated by faith healers, traditional medicine, in addition to modern psychiatry [38]. It is important to be aware of tradition and faith beliefs, and to incorporate them as much as possible in management plans in order to facilitate adherence to treatment.

3.4. Neurocognitive Disorders

Dementias are a group of diagnoses characterized by substantial decline from a previous level of functioning in at least one cognitive domain (complex attention, executive function, learning and memory, language, perceptual–motor, or social cognition) with loss of independence in activities of daily living. Criteria for the diagnosis of dementia are included in the Diagnostic and Statistics Manual, Fifth Revision (DSM-5). The most common dementia is Alzheimer's Dementia (AD), followed by Lewy body dementia and Vascular Dementia. Global estimates suggest that by 2040, over 71% of people living with dementia worldwide will reside in low- and middle-income countries, especially in sub-Saharan Africa [39]. The number of new cases anticipated each year worldwide is almost 7.7 million, of which 0.5 million is in Africa [40].

The report of the National Institute of Neurological and Communicative Disorders and Stroke and the Alzheimer's Disease and Related Disorders Association (NINCDS-ADRDA) Work Group under the Department of Health and Human Services Task Force on Alzheimer's disease established criteria for the definite, probable, possible, and unlikely AD. This is a clinical diagnosis, in which clinicians can make a diagnosis of AD and exclude other causes of dementia. In the United States, AD is also disproportionately high amongst African Americans. A growing body of evidence suggests that the prevalence of cognitive impairment or Alzheimer's disease may be two to three times higher among older African Americans than in older non-Hispanic whites. African Americans also carry a heavy burden with diabetes, obesity and other cardiovascular risk factors that are risk factors for vascular dementia as well as AD [41].

As with other mental illnesses, African Americans are underrepresented in clinical trials of dementia due to various barriers to recruitment and therefore makes it difficult to provide accurate estimates of prevalence.

Identification and intervention for Alzheimer's disease among blacks also remains challenging. Performance on cognitive function tests is still the gold standard for diagnosing Alzheimer's disease. However, education is closely tied to performance on these tests, and both years and quality of education tend to be lower in racial and ethnic minorities which creates serious challenges for accurate diagnoses in these populations. Screening tools commonly used for cognitive testing are the Alzheimer's Disease Assessment Scale-Cognitive Subscale (ADAS-Cog), Montreal Cognitive Assessment (MOCA), Mini Mental State Exam (MMSE), and Blessed Dementia Scale (BDS). Literacy levels greatly influence performance on tests. A study on low literacy groups in sub-Saharan Africa validated the use of ADAs-Cog for dementia screening [42]. The IDEA (Identification and Intervention for Dementia in Elderly Africans) screening tool has also been a valuable cognitive screen for use in populations of lower formal education. In one study, the Consortium to Establish a Registry for Alzheimer's disease (CERAD) total score and the Informant Questionnaire on Cognitive Decline in the Elderly (IQCODE) were used to assess cognitive performance and reported cognitive decline. A higher CERAD total score was associated with lower odds of cognitive impairment, no dementia (CIND) and dementia, at comparable ratios between African Americans and whites. Higher IQCODE scores were associated with increased odds of dementia in both African Americans and whites [43].

In addition to memory and other cognitive deficits, the broader effects of dementia include undernutrition, poor healthcare in general, and increased mortality (2.5 times) in older adults with dementia as compared to those without dementia. Decline in body mass index appears to be an early marker for dementia [44]. In a recent meta –analysis of studies on dementia, there was consistent evidence (mostly from the United States) that minority ethnic people access diagnostic services later in their illness and were also less likely to access anti-dementia medications, research trials, and 24-hour care upon receiving a diagnosis. African Americans were 30% less likely to be prescribed cholinesterase inhibitors [45].

Keeping in mind the growing number of blacks that will develop dementia in the next decades, a high degree of vigilance should include use of cognitive screening tools, encouragement towards acceptance of clinical trials, use of anti-dementia medications, treatment of the neuropsychiatric symptoms, and use of social community services. These should take priority for all healthcare providers in settings where the older black patients present for care. It is important that clinicians make a concerted effort to minimize false positive diagnoses as individuals suffer needlessly when falsely diagnosed with dementia. On the other hand, it is important that dementia be detected early. If dementia has progressed before an accurate diagnosis is made, individuals will have missed the opportunity to delay the progression of the disease through medication and other cognitive interventions [46].

Treatment for dementia includes prevention, harm reduction, mitigation, management of neuropsychiatric symptoms and social factors. Primary prevention starts with attention to nutrition, counseling, exercise, and regular screening for dementia. Secondary prevention focuses on optimum management of metabolic factors and treatment of hypertension [47], diabetes, and cardiovascular issues. Tertiary care is focused on, but not limited to, the use of medications. Medications used primarily include cholinesterase inhibitors and memantine. Drugs which aim to target the amyloid deposition on the brain are also under investigation.

Cholinesterase inhibitors such as donepezil, rivastigmine, and galantamine increase acetylcholine levels and have been approved by the U.S. Food and Drug Administration (FDA) for the treatment of AD. These are approved for all stages of dementia. The N-methyl-D-aspartate (NMDA)-receptor antagonist memantine is also approved for moderate to severe dementia. Donepezil, in a study in African Americans, was found to be safe and effective in this population [48].

The most frequent reason for hospitalizations or placement in nursing homes for patients with dementia are neuropsychiatric symptoms that occur almost universally. These include psychosis, agitation, apathy, depression, anxiety, disinhibition and other behavioral disturbances; all of which significantly affect quality of life.

Neuropsychiatric symptoms of dementia are very prevalent. A study in Central Africa and Congo showed 89.9% prevalence of this behavior [49] Some symptoms like depression and anxiety are more common in the early stages and other symptoms like hallucinations and delusions more common in the late stages, but do not necessarily follow a specific course. The Neuropsychiatric Inventory (NPI) is a good screening tool for evaluation of these symptoms. Depending on the particular symptom; antidepressant, antianxiety and antipsychotic medications can all be helpful. All should be used judiciously while keeping in mind comorbidities and interactions with other medications. The black box warning for use of antipsychotics in dementia patients should be carefully considered. Medications should ideally be used in collaboration with a multidisciplinary team that includes the patient's neurologist, psychiatrist and primary care provider. Regular reassessments for continuing use should also be performed.

Vascular dementia/Vascular neurocognitive disorder is the second most common form of dementia, accounting for almost 15% of dementias. African Americans have a higher rate of vascular dementia [50]. The risk factors for vascular dementia (including hypertension, diabetes, obesity and hyperlipidemia) are highly prevalent in the older black population and may contribute to this risk [47, 51, 52]. Screening and treating the risk factors may reduce the risk of dementia in this population [47].

The third most common form of dementia is Lewy Body dementia (LBD), more recently recognized as Neurocognitive Disorders with Lewy Bodies. However, there is very little information on this condition in African Americans specifically. The three core diagnostic criteria for LBD are fluctuating cognition, fluctuating alertness and attention, and recurrent, detailed, well-formed visual hallucinations. LBD is also associated with features of parkinsonism, which develop soon after cognitive decline. When LBD presents with psychosis, it is essential to remember the extreme sensitivity to neuroleptics. Severe and often fatal neuroleptic sensitivity may occur in older adult patients with confusion, dementia, or behavioral disturbance [53].

References

[1] Taylor RJ, Chatters LM. Psychiatric disorders among older Black Americans: within-and between-group differences. *Innov Aging.* 2020; 4(3):igaa007.

[2] Ford BC, Bullard KM, Taylor RJ, Toler AK, Neighbors HW, Jackson JS. Lifetime and 12-month prevalence of Diagnostic and Statistical

Manual of Mental Disorders, Fourth Edition disorders among older African Americans: findings from the National Survey of American Life. *Am J Geriatr Psychiatry Off J Am Assoc Geriatr Psychiatry.* 2007; 15(8):652-659.

[3] Woodward AT, Taylor RJ, Abelson JM, Matusko N. Major depressive disorder among older African Americans, Caribbean blacks, and non-Hispanic whites: secondary analysis of the National Survey of American Life. *Depress Anxiety*. 2013; 30(6):589-597.

[4] Joe S, Ford BC, Taylor RJ, Chatters LM. Prevalence of suicide ideation and attempts among Black Americans in later life. *Transcult Psychiatry*. 2014; 51(2):190-208.

[5] Akinyemi E, Watkins DC, Kavanagh J, Johnson-Lawrence V, Lynn S, Kales HC. A qualitative comparison of DSM depression criteria to language used by older church-going African-Americans. *Aging Ment Health*. 2018; 22(9):1149-1155.

[6] Tollman SM, Salomon JA, Geldsetzer P, et al. Depressive Symptoms and Their Relation to Age and Chronic Diseases Among Middle-Aged and Older Adults in Rural South Africa. *J Gerontol A Biol Sci Med Sci*. 2019; 74(6).

[7] Gallo JJ, Cooper-Patrick L, Lesikar S. Depressive symptoms of whites and African Americans aged 60 years and older. *J Gerontol B Psychol Sci Soc Sci*. 1998; 53(5):P277-286.

[8] Baker FM, Okwumabua J, Philipose V, Wong S. Screening African-American elderly for the presence of depressive symptoms: a preliminary investigation. *J Geriatr Psychiatry Neurol.* 1996; 9(3): 127-132.

[9] Mills TL, Alea NL, Cheong JA. Differences in the indicators of depressive symptoms among a community sample of African-American and Caucasian older adults. *Community Ment Health J.* 2004; 40(4):309-331.

[10] Pickett YR, Bazelais KN, Bruce ML. Late-life depression in older African Americans: a comprehensive review of epidemiological and clinical data. *Int J Geriatr Psychiatry*. 2013; 28(9):903-913.

[11] Naidoo I, Charlton KE, Esterhuizen T, Cassim B, Esterhuizen TM. High risk of malnutrition associated with depressive symptoms in older South Africans living in KwaZulu-Natal, South Africa: a cross-sectional survey. *J Health Popul Nutr*. 2015; 33.

[12] Ward EC, Mengesha MM, Issa F. Older African American women's lived experiences with depression and coping behaviours. *J Psychiatr Ment Health Nurs*. 2014; 21(1):46-59.

[13] Cornish EK, Bergner EM, Griffith DM. "They have said that I was slightly depressed but there are circumstances that bring that on": How Middle-Aged and Older African American Men Describe Perceived Stress and Depression. *Ethn Dis*. 2017; 27(4):437-442.

[14] Gitlin LN, Chernett NL, Dennis MP, Hauck WW. Identification of and beliefs about depressive symptoms and preferred treatment approaches among community-living older African Americans. *Am J Geriatr Psychiatry Off J Am Assoc Geriatr Psychiatry*. 2012; 20(11):973-984.

[15] Jeffrey M, Diah KC, Capp K, Stripling A. The Geriatric Depression Scale - Short Form (GDS - SF): A Model For African American Populations. *Gerontologist.* 2016; 56. Accessed October 19, 2020. https://proxy01.its.virginia.edu/login?url=https://search.ebscohost.com/login.aspx?direct=true&site=eds-live&db=edswss&AN=000388585001666.

[16] Pedraza O, Dotson VM, Willis FB, Graff-Radford NR, Lucas JA. Internal Consistency and Test-Retest Stability of the Geriatric Depression Scale-Short Form in African American Older Adults. *J Psychopathol Behav Assess*. 2009; 31(4):412-416.

[17] Coman EN, Iordache E, Schensul JJ, Coiculescu I. Comparisons of CES-D depression scoring methods in two older adults ethnic groups. The emergence of an ethnic-specific brief three-item CES-D scale. *Int J Geriatr Psychiatry*. 2013; 28(4):424-432.

[18] Li C, Friedman B, Conwell Y, Fiscella K. Validity of the Patient Health Questionnaire 2 (PHQ-2) in identifying major depression in older people. *J Am Geriatr Soc*. 2007; 55(4):596-602.

[19] Case BG, Bertollo DN, Laska EM, Siegel CE, Wanderling JA, Olfson M. Racial differences in the availability and use of electroconvulsive

therapy for recurrent major depression. *J Affect Disord.* 2012; 136(3):359-365.

[20] Jones KC, Salemi JL, Dongarwar D, et al. Racial/Ethnic Disparities in Receipt of Electroconvulsive Therapy for Elderly Patients With a Principal Diagnosis of Depression in Inpatient Settings. *Am J Geriatr Psychiatry Off J Am Assoc Geriatr Psychiatry.* 2019; 27(3):266-278.

[21] Olagunju AT, Olutoki MO, Ogunnubi OP, Adeyemi JD. Late-life depression: Burden, severity and relationship with social support dimensions in a West African community. *Arch Gerontol Geriatr.* 2015; 61(2).

[22] Schubert JR, Coles ME, Heimberg RG, Weiss BD. Disseminating treatment for anxiety disorders step 2: peer recommendations to seek help. *J Anxiety Disord.* 2014; 28(7):712-716.

[23] Ostir GV, Goodwin JS. High anxiety is associated with an increased risk of death in an older tri-ethnic population. *J Clin Epidemiol.* 2006; 59(5):534-540.

[24] Kim YA, Morales KH, Bogner HR. Patient ethnicity and the identification of anxiety in elderly primary care patients. *J Am Geriatr Soc.* 2008; 56(9):1626-1630.

[25] Taylor DJ, Lichstein KL, Durrence HH, Reidel BW, Bush AJ. Epidemiology of insomnia, depression, and anxiety. *Sleep.* 2005; 28(11):1457-1464.

[26] Cohen CI, Magai C, Yaffee R, Walcott-Brown L. The prevalence of anxiety and associated factors in a multiracial sample of older adults. *Psychiatr Serv Wash DC.* 2006; 57(12):1719-1725.

[27] Williams MT, Domanico J, Marques L, Leblanc NJ, Turkheimer E. Barriers to treatment among African Americans with obsessive-compulsive disorder. *J Anxiety Disord.* 2012; 26(4):555-563.

[28] Jameson JP, Shrestha S, Escamilla M, et al. Establishing community partnerships to support late-life anxiety research: lessons learned from the Calmer Life project. *Aging Ment Health.* 2012; 16(7):874-883.

[29] Bashir M, Holroyd S. Caring for the elderly female psychiatric patient. *Psychiatr Clin North Am.* 2010; 33(2):475-485.

[30] Qassem T, Bebbington P, Spiers N, McManus S, Jenkins R, Dein S. Prevalence of psychosis in black ethnic minorities in Britain: analysis based on three national surveys. *Soc Psychiatry Psychiatr Epidemiol.* 2015; 50(7):1057-1064.

[31] Earl TR, Fortuna LR, Gao S, et al. An exploration of how psychotic-like symptoms are experienced, endorsed, and understood from the National Latino and Asian American Study and National Survey of American Life. *Ethn Health.* 2015; 20(3):273-292.

[32] Reinhardt MM, Cohen CI. Late-life psychosis: diagnosis and treatment. *Curr Psychiatry Rep.* 2015; 17(2):1.

[33] Howard R, Rabins PV, Seeman MV, Jeste DV. Late-onset schizophrenia and very-late-onset schizophrenia-like psychosis: an international consensus. The International Late-Onset Schizophrenia Group. *Am J Psychiatry.* 2000; 157(2):172-178.

[34] Tisher A, Salardini A. A Comprehensive Update on Treatment of Dementia. *Semin Neurol.* 2019; 39(2):167-178.

[35] D'Souza C, Gupta A, Alldrick MD, Sastry BS. Management of psychosis in Parkinson's disease. *Int J Clin Pract.* 2003; 57(4):295-300.

[36] Hanagasi HA, Emre M. Treatment of behavioural symptoms and dementia in Parkinson's disease. *Fundam Clin Pharmacol.* 2005; 19(2):133-146.

[37] Lawson WB, Herman BK, Loebel A, Lazariciu I, Malik M. Ziprasidone in Black patients with schizophrenia: analysis of four short-term, double-blind studies. *CNS Spectr.* 2009; 14(9):478-486.

[38] Chidarikire S, Cross M, Skinner I, Cleary M. Treatments for people living with schizophrenia in Sub-Saharan Africa: an adapted realist review. *Int Nurs Rev.* 2018; 65(1):78-92.

[39] Ojagbemi A, Daley S. Implementing the Dementia Carers Support Initiative of the National Institute for Health and Care Excellence in a sub-Saharan African Setting. *J Health Care Poor Underserved.* 2015; 26(4).

[40] Brito-Aguilar R. Dementia Around the World and the Latin America and Mexican Scenarios. *J Alzheimers Dis JAD.* 2019; 71(1):1-5.

[41] Obisesan TO, Gillum RF, Johnson S, et al. Neuroprotection and neurodegeneration in Alzheimer's disease: role of cardiovascular disease risk factors, implications for dementia rates, and prevention with aerobic exercise in african americans. *Int J Alzheimers Dis.* 2012; 2012:568382.

[42] Paddick S-M, Kisoli A, Mkenda S, et al. Adaptation and validation of the Alzheimer's Disease Assessment Scale - Cognitive (ADAS-Cog) in a low-literacy setting in sub-Saharan Africa. *Acta Neuropsychiatr.* 2017; 29(4).

[43] Potter GG, Plassman BL, Burke JR, et al. Cognitive performance and informant reports in the diagnosis of cognitive impairment and dementia in African Americans and whites. *Alzheimers Dement J Alzheimers Assoc.* 2009; 5(6):445-453.

[44] Gao S, Nguyen JT, Hendrie HC, et al. Accelerated weight loss and incident dementia in an elderly African-American cohort. *J Am Geriatr Soc.* 2011; 59(1):18-25.

[45] Cooper C, Tandy AR, Balamurali TBS, Livingston G. A systematic review and meta-analysis of ethnic differences in use of dementia treatment, care, and research. *Am J Geriatr Psychiatry Off J Am Assoc Geriatr Psychiatry.* 2010; 18(3):193-203.

[46] Black S, Simpson GM. *A Call to Action: Dementia Screening of Alzheimer's Disease in Older African Americans.* Vol 9. (Vakalahi HFO, Simpson GM, Giunta N, eds.). Springer; 2014:229-238.

[47] Welsh T, Masoli J. Antihypertensive medications may reduce the risk of dementia in older African-Americans with hypertension. *Evid Based Nurs.* 2018; 21(4):104.

[48] Griffith P, Lichtenberg P, Goldman R, Payne-Parrish J. Safety and efficacy of donepezil in African Americans with mild-to-moderate Alzheimer's disease. *J Natl Med Assoc.* 2006; 98(10):1590-1597.

[49] Yoro-Zohoun I, Houinato D, Nubukpo P, et al. Severity of Neuropsychiatric Symptoms and Distress in Dementia among Older People in Central Africa (EPIDEMCA Study). *J Am Geriatr Soc.* 2020; 68(1).

Africa, this cost is usually borne by the extended family who provide support for the affected individual. As a result of this, it is difficult to quantify the cost of the disabilities for the most part.

2. Clinical Diseases

2.1. Osteoarthritis

Osteoarthritis (OA) is the most common form of arthritis and is a heterogeneous group of conditions with varying degrees of disease manifestation. The majority of patients present with joint pain and functional limitations [4], but the age of disease onset, sequence of joint involvement, and disease progression vary in different individuals. Older adults are the most affected by OA. The condition ranges from an asymptomatic, incidental finding on clinical or radiologic examination to a progressive disabling disorder that can ultimately lead to 'joint failure.'

2.1.1. Prevalence

Worldwide, it is estimated that about 240 million people are affected by OA [5], including over 30 million in the United States. This increased from 21 million in 1990 and 27 million in 2005 [6]. There is a relative paucity of statistics concerning the prevalence of OA on the African continent. The global prevalence of hip and knee OA approximates 5 percent in adults over 18 years of age, taking into account differences between rural and urban areas, and between high and low to moderate income regions. This rate will likely climb up as the population ages and obesity rates go up [4]. The prevalence of OA increases with age, with just under 10 percent of men and 18 percent of women over the age of 60 years reporting symptomatic OA [7].

2.1.2. Clinical Presentation

Osteoarthritis affects specific joints such as knees, hips, interphalangeal joints, and first carpometacarpal joints. The majority of patients develop symptoms in their middle or older age. 'Wear and tear' related joint pain, the 'gelling' phenomenon with short-lived morning stiffness or joint stiffness after periods of prolonged inactivity, and locomotor restriction are common presenting symptoms. Movement induced pain and joint line tenderness may be elicited in early disease. The presence of crepitus, bony enlargement, and a reduced range of movement may be seen in more advanced cases. More severe cases of OA are characterized by rest pain, night pain, sarcopenia and deformity. The cardinal features of inflammation are usually absent. However, mild to moderate effusions may be found in the knee joint. The diagnosis of OA can be made on clinical grounds alone when the classic symptoms and signs are elicited. Imaging studies may show changes of OA, but generally there is a discordance between the symptoms, signs, radiographic changes, and disability in OA [8].

2.1.3. Specific Disease Characteristics in Africa

There is a preponderance of infections such as Tuberculosis and HIV in Africa which can affect joints directly and indirectly leading to alterations in joint anatomy with the subsequent development of osteoarthritis [9]. A significant percentage of the population in rural areas engage in physically taxing work thereby increasing the risk of joint injury and/or overload. These increase the risk of developing osteoarthritis significantly.

2.1.4. Clinical Management

The goals of treatment are to decrease joint pain and stiffness; to increase joint mobility and muscle strength; improve the quality of life for the patient(s). There are different modalities of treatment including medications, physical and occupational therapy, non-surgical therapies and surgery. Alternative therapies are also available with varying degrees of success. Osteoarthritis lacks the broad array of medications that are available to treat most other forms of arthritis. This limitation notwithstanding, there are still options to choose from including prescription and non-prescription options. Medications include Acetaminophen, Non-steroidal anti-inflammatory drugs (NSAIDs) and Duloxetine. Physical therapy is helpful in improving the range of mobility and increasing muscle strength. Occupational therapy is helpful in guiding affected individuals to adapt to their surrounding environment. Weight loss is appropriate in those who are overweight or obese. Intra-articular injections of steroid and/or hyaluronic acid have been found useful by many patients. Surgical procedures are usually an option of last resort. Surgical procedures that can be carried out include osteotomies, partial and total joint replacements. Alternative therapies such as ginger, black pepper, turmeric, glucosamine, chondroitin and methylsulfonylmethane (MSM) have all been reported to be helpful in reducing the level of pain by many patients [4, 8].

2.2. Low Back Pain

2.2.1. Prevalence

Low back pain (LBP) is a common condition affecting many individuals at some point in their lives. It is not a disease in the strictest sense but is a very common symptom occurring secondary to various conditions. The incidence increases with age. It is estimated that between 5 to 10% of people with low back pain will go on to have chronic low back pain. This leads to high treatment costs, the loss of income, and individual suffering, in addition to being one of the main reasons for people to seek health care services. Although chronic low back pain is highly disabling, information about its prevalence and associated factors are haphazardly found in medical literature. Most results are presented in a secondary manner in studies evaluating several musculoskeletal outcomes simultaneously [10]. An example is of a cross-sectional study in a rural hospital in south-western Nigeria examining the prevalence of low back pain among its staff. Seventy four out of eighty staff members at the facility participated in the study. The overall prevalence of low back pain was 46%. The highest prevalence of back pain (69%) was recorded among nursing staff, followed by administrative staff (55%) and custodial staff (47%). Heavy physical work

(45%), poor posture (20%) and prolonged standing or sitting (20%) were the most frequent activities reported to be associated with low back pain among staff members. The prevalence of low back pain among these staff members is comparable to those in higher income countries. Health education on posture and correct lifting techniques may reduce the burden of low back pain [11].

2.2.2. Clinical Presentation

There are several causes of low back pain with varying clinical presentations depending on the underlying cause of pain. The various causes can be grouped broadly into mechanical low back pain, non-mechanical spine disease and visceral organ disease. Mechanical low back pain refers to back pain that arises intrinsically from the spine, intervertebral disks, or surrounding soft tissues. This includes lumbosacral muscle strain, disc herniation, lumbar spondylosis, spondylolisthesis, spondylolysis, vertebral compression fractures, and acute or chronic traumatic injury. Overuse and recurrent trauma are common causes of chronic mechanical low back pain. These can frequently be observed with workplace injuries. Many individuals who experience activity-limiting low back pain will go on to experience recurrent episodes. Chronic low back pain affects up to 23% of the population worldwide, with an estimated 24% to 80% of patients having a recurrence at one year [12]. There are relatively fewer studies out of Africa on this topic. A recent systematic review of thirty-four studies estimates the annual prevalence of LBP in Africa at 57% (95% CI: 51-63) [13].

Non mechanical spine diseases leading to the development of low back pain include neoplasia (multiple myeloma, metastatic carcinoma, lymphoma, leukemia, spinal cord tumors and retro-peritoneal tumors), infection (osteomyelitis, septic discitis, para-spinous abscess, and epidural abscess), inflammatory arthritis (ankylosing spondylitis, psoriatic spondylitis, reactive arthritis, and inflammatory bowel disease), Scheuermann disease and Paget disease [14].

Visceral diseases that can cause back pain include those of pelvic organs (prostatitis, endometriosis, and chronic pelvic inflammatory disease), renal disease (nephrolithiasis, pyelonephritis, and perinephric abscess), aortic aneurysm, gastrointestinal disease (pancreatitis, cholecystitis, and penetrating ulcer) and fat herniation of lumbar space.

2.2.3. Specific Disease Characteristics in Africa

Many older African adults performed physically challenging work in their younger years. This clearly takes a toll on their bodies. A very interesting finding on a review of literature regarding low back pain in older African adults clearly showed a notable difference in point and annual low back pain prevalence of almost 20% between males and females, with males reporting a higher prevalence [15]. These results indicate a reverse gender pattern compared to global trends which generally indicate that females experience a higher prevalence of low back pain. The intriguing aspect of this finding is that within most African cultures, African males actually tend to under-report health issues, as many men fear that admitting to having health issues makes one to be thought of as less masculine. One would therefore expect a higher prevalence of low back pain for African females. The studies looked at individuals mostly in industrial work settings and may not be generalizable to the general population.

2.2.4. Clinical Management

The modalities of cognitive behavioral therapy (CBT) and physical therapy may offer the best potential for relief from low back pain. Drug therapy frequently offers temporary relief, especially for acute back pain. These are however, not usually beneficial in people with chronic back pain. Acetaminophen (also known as paracetamol in Europe and many African countries) and non-steroidal anti-inflammatory drugs (NSAIDS) bring the pain to a tolerable level. These medications are not designed for more than a few days of use at a time. They are preferred as first-line medications for acute non-radicular back pain. Using patient-specific risk factors and prior response to medication therapy may help determine the choice of medications. Opioid based medications, such as tramadol, may be used with caution and are for short term use only, as the risk of addiction increases with the length of therapy. Bed rest, supportive corsets, and braces no longer have a place in the management of low back pain. Corticosteroids may give transient relief and should be used with caution due to the associated risks. Tricyclic antidepressants in small doses can help with regulating the sleep cycle. Muscle relaxants may help in certain instances. Physical therapy, in addition to, chiropractic and other manipulative treatments may provide some pain relief, partly due to the comfort effect of touch and the amount of time that the affected individual gets to spend with the practitioner. These forms of therapy are not widely available and can be cost prohibitive.

2.3. Neck Pain

Neck pain is one of the most common debilitating musculoskeletal complaints affecting the older population. Low back pain and neck pain have been identified in recent years as the leading causes of disability. Neck pain is described as pain in the neck with or without referred pain into one or both upper limbs.

2.3.1. Prevalence

The annual prevalence of neck pain is about 30% – 50%, with a point prevalence of 4.7% and a lifetime prevalence of 14.2% – 70% worldwide [15]. The point prevalence of neck pain in the sub-Saharan Africa region is high (males 4.7%; females 6.7%), exceeded only by the United States (males 5.3%; females 7.6%), Western Europe (males 5.2%; females 7.4%) and East Asia (males 4.8%; females 7.0%). There was also a significant increase of neck pain prevalence between 1990 and 2015 [17]. Possible reasons cited for the increase in neck pain are an ageing population and increasing obesity. From estimates for the global burden of neck pain (2000–2010), it was found that neck pain is more prevalent in women compared to men and peaks between 40 and 50 years of age [16].

2.3.2. Clinical Presentation

The main symptom is pain in the cervical region radiating to the occiput, neck muscles, shoulders and upper limbs. The presence of retro-orbital and/or temporal pain suggests referral from the upper cervical levels. This can mimic giant cell arteritis. Some patients develop anterior chest pain, which may resemble coronary ischemia. Stiffness may be reversible or irreversible and is usually associated with pain. Numbness, tingling or weakness in the upper limbs when present, is ill-defined, unless there is nerve root entrapment when it can follow a radicular pattern. Dizziness or poor balance may result from vertebral artery involvement or irritation of the sympathetic nerves and is usually exacerbated by neck movement if this is the etiology. Other less common symptoms include dysphagia (due to large anterior osteophytes), dyspnea, or the triggering of a migraine headache [18].

The differential diagnoses to be considered in a patient presenting with neck pain should include: soft tissue lesions (acute neck strain, acute torticollis), fibromyalgia and psychogenic causes, mechanical lesions [disc prolapse, diffuse idiopathic skeletal hyperostosis (DISH)], inflammatory (rheumatoid, ankylosing spondylitis, polymyalgia rheumatica), metabolic (Paget's disease, osteoporosis, gout, pseudo-gout), infective (osteomyelitis, tuberculosis), malignancy (primary tumors, secondary deposits, myeloma) and adjacent pathology (shoulder or acromioclavicular disease).

2.3.3. Specific Disease Characteristics in Africa

There are more females than males who complain of having neck pain in Africa. Many females are compelled to carry weights on their heads from a relatively young age and this puts them at increased risk of developing neck pain from various ailments.

2.3.4. Clinical Management

The initial treatment for all patients with acute neck pain includes patient education, postural modification, early mobilization through participation in a home exercise program, and treatment with pain medications, if needed. For patients whose neck pain has resolved, they need to be encouraged to adhere to recommendations regarding proper posture and sleep position. Continued participation with the home exercises is also important to reduce symptom recurrence.

Patient education and reassurance is crucial in helping the patient understand that the condition is common, the natural history of the condition, the prognosis of the condition and the importance maintaining physical fitness, proper posture, ergonomics and regular, sufficient sleep.

Posture and sleep position modifications are useful. Posture modifications to correct muscle tension are an essential part of the treatment regimen for neck pain and include sitting straight with the crown of the head tall, chin minimally tilted down, shoulders down, and the scapula retracted and depressed. Recognizing and adopting a neutral posture and engaging in a natural, regular breathing pattern may allow the patient to correct contributors to neck muscle tension. Avoiding a sustained or prolonged seated position is beneficial. Patients should make an effort to stand and walk frequently during the day and perform cervical range of motion exercises while at work. The avoidance of carrying heavy loads is recommended to help relieve and prevent the recurrence of acute neck pain. The head and neck should be aligned with the body when sleeping. A preferred sleep position is to have the patient lie flat on their back with thighs elevated on pillows with a relatively small pillow under the head and neck, thereby flattening the long spinal muscles. For side sleepers, use of a slightly larger pillow may help maintain proper cervical spine alignment.

Early mobilization with participation in a home exercise program helps patients maintain cervical range of motion and encourages them to become active participants in their own care. The exercises taught are gentle stretching exercises that should be performed on a daily basis as tolerated. These include neck rotation, neck tilting, neck bending, shoulder rolls, scapular retraction, deep neck flexor strengthening, and anterior chest wall stretches. Before each exercise session, patients are advised to warm their neck and upper back muscles. This can be achieved with warm compresses or a warm bath. The muscles should be gently stretched in sets of 10 to 15 repetitions as tolerated. It is best to perform the exercises at least twice daily: in the morning and just before bedtime. For those patients whose pain has resolved, the home exercise program should be continued to maintain neck range of motion and flexibility. The use of topical heat or cold may help with the short-term pain relief in some patients with acute neck pain. The modalities of heat or cold can be applied every two to three hours as needed. Adjunctive pharmacologic therapy is reserved for patients with acute neck pain who are experiencing significant discomfort. This is useful for additional symptom management when non-pharmacologic therapy, which is generally preferred over pharmacologic therapy has not been effective. However, both modalities are frequently used together. The aim of introducing pharmacologic therapy is to provide relief of pain symptoms while allowing the patient to participate in a home exercise program. The preferred first-line medications are nonsteroidal anti-inflammatory drug (NSAID) or acetaminophen as pharmacotherapy for acute non-radicular neck pain. Using patient-specific risk factors and prior response to medication therapy help determine which one to use first. NSAIDs are associated with possible gastrointestinal, kidney, and cardiovascular side effects; risk factors for complications from NSAID therapy should be assessed before prescribing these medications. For patients who have previously tried an NSAID with good pain relief, and who are not at increased risk from an NSAID-related complication, one of these can be used. Using the lowest effective dose for the shortest period of time should be an important consideration. Patients who are unable to take NSAIDs (for example due to allergy or other intolerance, chronic kidney disease, hypertension, peptic ulcer disease, or cardiovascular disease), or who have previously tried acetaminophen with good pain relief, this is the preferred option. A non-benzodiazepine skeletal muscle relaxant can be prescribed for symptoms not well managed with an NSAID or acetaminophen, especially for those with prominent muscle spasm. The medication should be ideally used at bedtime. The medication should be used for the shortest time possible.

For patients with acute non-radicular neck pain, for whom NSAID or acetaminophen with a skeletal muscle relaxant fails to adequately control pain symptoms, consideration should be given to adding a small dose of tramadol to their regimen. An alternative is to use tramadol in place of the skeletal muscle relaxant. The lowest possible dose of tramadol for the shortest period of time, should be used. The risk of sedation, especially when used with muscle relaxants needs to be emphasized.

2.4. Rheumatoid Arthritis

Rheumatoid arthritis (RA) is a chronic, systemic, inflammatory disorder of unknown etiology that primarily involves synovial joints. It has an autoimmune basis and the arthritis is typically symmetrical, and can lead, if not controlled, to destruction of joints due to erosion of cartilage and bone, causing joint deformities. The condition can result in significant locomotor disability within a decade or two, in patients who do not fully respond to treatment.

2.4.1. Prevalence

Over the last two decades, at least ten population-based studies have been conducted in Africa to determine the prevalence of RA in Africa. Generally speaking, there seems to be an increase in the prevalence of RA with urbanization. In view of the fact that the African continent is the fastest urbanizing continent, the numbers of RA will increase in future. No environmental factor was identified during these studies to explain this phenomenon. The "hygiene hypothesis" associated with the modern lifestyle, which suggests a connection between lower incidence of infections and higher rates of autoimmune disorders, may partly explain the phenomenon. The combined prevalence in Africa is said to be 0.7% which is lower than the estimated world prevalence of 1%. It should be kept in mind that the American College of Rheumatology (ACR) 1987 criteria was used in these studies, which is less sensitive than the newer 2010 ACR/European League against Rheumatism (ACR/EU- LAR) criteria [19].

2.4.2. Clinical Presentation

Rheumatoid arthritis has previously been uncommonly reported among Africans and rarely among West Africans [20]. Most reports were from Southern Africa. In recent years it has been found that rheumatoid arthritis is not uncommon in Africans. Rheumatoid arthritis (RA) most typically presents as polyarticular disease and with a gradual onset, but some patients can present with acute onset with intermittent or migratory joint involvement or with monoarticular disease. The features of early rheumatoid inflammation are pain and swelling of the affected joints. Inflammation with local tenderness from pressure applied on the joint or by pain on moving the joint. Swelling may be due to synovial hypertrophy or effusion. Heat and redness are not prominent features of RA, although an involved joint is frequently warmer than non-involved joints, if carefully examined. The classic joint deformities seen in RA are late manifestations of the disease that result from the physical stresses and damage to the local anatomy of involved joints. The arthritis can affect the patient's capacity to perform the activities of daily living, as well as, their ability to do their job. Systemic symptoms can also manifest in these patients. The systemic symptoms that may be present on evaluation include myalgia, fatigue, low-grade fever, weight loss, and depression. Other features that may be seen are rheumatoid nodules or eye involvement. RA onset is usually insidious, with joint pain, morning stiffness and joint swelling being prominent. Classically, the metacarpophalangeal (MCP) and proximal interphalangeal (PIP) joints of the fingers, the interphalangeal joints of the thumbs, the wrists, and the metatarsophalangeal (MTP) joints of the toes are sites of early involvement. Other synovial joints such as the elbows, shoulders, ankles, and knees can be affected. Morning stiffness is a common feature of those with active RA. The duration of the morning stiffness usually reflects the severity of joint inflammation.

2.4.3. Specific Disease Characteristics in Africa

The prevalence of tuberculosis (TB) is high in many parts of Africa. RA patients are at increased risk of TB due to drugs used to treat RA including glucocorticoids, methotrexate, and biologic drugs, in particular tumor necrosis factor inhibitor (anti-TNF) therapy. Each patient requires screening for latent tuberculosis infection (LTBI) and an assessment of the risk of TB infection/ reactivation. The burden of HIV infection is highest in the world in southern Africa, with an estimated 33% of females between the ages of 25 and 29 years infected in 2010. This pandemic has both diagnostic and therapeutic implications for the management of patients with concomitant inflammatory arthritis. HIV infection can cause, among other musculoskeletal syndromes, inflammatory polyarthritis mimicking RA. HIV testing may be appropriate in a patient presenting with inflammatory arthritis. There are several challenges in the management of RA patients who are HIV-positive. Information on the safety of using immunosuppressive drugs in an HIV-positive patient is limited. MTX and biologic drugs place patients at risk of opportunistic infections and there is concern of added immunosuppression if prescribed in an HIV-positive patient. For this reason, these therapies are not recommended and hydroxychloroquine (HCQ) and/or chloroquine (CQ) or sulfasalazine (SSZ) may be more appropriate choices for treatment. In addition, there are difficulties in the assessment of disease activity in HIV-positive patients due to the nonspecific increase in erythrocyte sedimentation rate (ESR) associated with HIV infection. Little is known about the effect of antiretroviral therapy (ART) on RA disease, or the safety of biologic drugs in patients receiving ART. These are areas for future research [19].

2.4.4. Clinical Management

Treatment guidelines recommend a treat-to-target of low disease activity or remission according to a validated disease activity measure [21–23]. Several measures have been developed and validated for use in clinical care to assess RA activity and aid in treatment decisions. The four most commonly used measures are Disease activity score (DAS28), Clinical disease activity index (CDAI), Simple disease activity index (SDAI) and Routine assessment of patient index data 3 (RAPID3). Their components are; number of tender joints, number of swollen joints, physician global assessment (0–10), laboratory tests: ESR or C - reactive protein (CRP), patient global assessment (0–10), patient function and patient pain.

Methotrexate (MTX) is the most widely prescribed disease modifying anti-rheumatic drug (DMARD). It is the gold standard of RA treatment. It is recommended as first-line therapy with rapid dose escalation according to response and tolerability to a maximum of 25 mg weekly. The drug has an excellent safety profile. Mild elevation of liver enzymes is not infrequent but usually transient, and cirrhosis is rare. There is no evidence that doses higher than 25 mg weekly are more effective and they may increase toxicity. The antimalarial (chloroquine [CQ]) or hydroxychloroquine (HCQ), may be used as monotherapy for mild RA, or in combination with MTX for moderate to severe disease. Sulfasalazine (SSZ) is effective as monotherapy and is particularly useful in patients in whom CQ, hydroxychloroquine and MTX are contraindicated. It can also be used in combination DMARD therapy. Leflunomide may be prescribed as monotherapy or co-prescribed with MTX. Patients who have failed MTX monotherapy should be treated with combination synthetic DMARDs. The most commonly prescribed combination treatment is MTX, SSZ, and CQ/HCQ. Glucocorticoids (GCs) rapidly reduce symptoms of RA and may inhibit development of erosions, particularly in early RA when used in combination with DMARDs. Potential side-effects make long-term use, undesirable. Low dose oral GC therapy is appropriate in combination with DMARDs in the treatment of early RA for up to 6 months. In established RA, they may be used as 'bridging' therapy when DMARDs are initiated. The GC therapy should be withdrawn once DMARDs have controlled the disease. Intra-articular GCs are useful for a mono- or oligo-articular flare of disease. Long-acting intramuscular methylprednisolone may be used as an alternative to oral prednisone. One of the most significant advances in the treatment of RA in recent years has been the development of biologic DMARDs, which are proteins directed against specific cytokines or their cell receptors. A broad array of biologic DMARDs are available. These have proven to be very effective in controlling RA in patients who have failed synthetic DMARD therapy with improvement of physical function and health-related quality of life. They may be classified into those inhibiting tumor necrosis factor (anti-TNF) and those targeting other cytokines or cells (non-anti-TNF). Biologic DMARDs are usually co-prescribed with MTX to improve efficacy. The introduction of biologic therapy should be considered in very severe cases and also after a trial period of at least 6 months on three synthetic DMARDs has not worked. Indications for biologic therapy include an inadequate response to synthetic DMARD therapy, with high disease activity (SDAI > 26), or moderate disease activity (SDAI 11 to 26) in the presence of poor prognostic factors (seropositivity, radiographic erosions within the first 2 years, extra-articular complications or functional disability). The efficacy of all currently available biologic drugs has been confirmed by clinical trials and by clinical experience. Drug choice depends on the safety profile and on the patient's preferred route of administration.

2.5. Gout

Gout is a chronic joint disease with deposition of monosodium urate crystals (MSU), which form in the presence of increased urate concentrations. Although environmental factors contribute to hyperuricemia, renal and gut excretion of urate is central to regulation of serum urate, as well as genetic factors. Activation of the NLRP3 inflammasome and release of interleukin 1β have key roles in initiation of acute gout flares. A "treat to target serum urate" approach is essential for effective gout management; long-term lowering of serum urate to less than 360μmol/L (6mg/dL) leads to crystal dissolution and ultimately to suppression of flares. An allopurinol dose-escalation strategy is frequently effective for achieving treatment targets, and several new urate-lowering drugs are also available. Worldwide, rates of initiation and continuation of urate-lowering therapy are very low, and, consequently, achievement of serum urate targets is infrequent [24].

2.5.1. Prevalence

There is a paucity of studies on the prevalence of gout in Africa. It is thought that the incidence and prevalence of gout in Africa mirror what is found elsewhere around the world. In Burkina Faso, a hospital-based study found gout prevalence of 0.30% (95%CI: 0.30 to 0.90) among HIV-infected patients undergoing antiretroviral therapy [25].

2.5.2. Clinical Presentation

Gout classically presents for the first time as an acute episode of inflammation affecting the foot or ankle. The most common site of involvement is the first metatarsophalangeal joint. The first flare often occurs after an asymptomatic period of hyperuricemia. It is self-limiting with complete resolution in signs and symptoms within a few days. If hyperuricemia persists, recurrent flares can occur, which become increasingly frequent and prolonged and affect many joints (polyarticular flares), including joints of the upper limbs. When hyperuricemia remains untreated, advanced gout with tophi or chronic gouty arthritis, or both, can develop in some individuals. Advanced gout is characterized by chronic joint pain, activity limitation, structural joint damage, and frequent flares. Gout has an important effect on musculoskeletal function and health-related quality of life, particularly in patients with frequent flares and tophaceous disease. Poorly controlled gout leads to absences from work, health-care use, and reduced social participation. Comorbid disorders can further contribute to poor health-related quality of life in people with gout.

2.5.3. Specific Disease Characteristics in Africa

There are some unique presentations of gout in the African continent associated with HIV disease. Before the introduction of HAART, the mortality rates from HIV were high, but with better care, patients now live longer, and there is a rise in cardio-metabolic disease among HIV patients. Protease inhibitors are associated with hyperuricemia. Other unique associations include vertigo and sickle cell anemia [26].

2.5.4. Clinical Management

Gout management includes rapid treatment of acute flares and effective long-term management. The central strategy for long-term management is reduction of serum urate to a concentration that achieves dissolution of monosodium urate crystals. The American College of Rheumatology guidelines state that urate-lowering therapy is indicated for those with recurrent gout flares (more than one flare a year), tophi, stage 2 or worse chronic kidney disease, or kidney stones. Urate-lowering therapy is not recommended for people with asymptomatic hyperuricemia. For patients with gout commencing urate-lowering therapy, selecting a target serum urate concentration dependent on disease severity of the individual patient, is important. The American College of Rheumatology guidelines recommend a target serum urate of less than 360 μmol/L (6 mg/dL) for all patients on urate-lowering therapy. Prolonged lowering of serum urate concentrations to less than this cutoff leads to dissolution of monosodium urate crystals, suppression of flares, and regression of tophi. A lower target of less than 300 μmol/L (5mg/dL) is recommended for patients with tophaceous or severe disease, as this concentration is associated with more rapid tophus regression. Traditionally, urate-lowering therapy is commenced at least 2 weeks after an acute flare. However, two recent studies [27] have shown that starting urate-lowering therapy during a gout flare does not prolong the flare, provided that the acute episode is adequately treated. When indicated, urate-lowering therapy should be started, and serum urate monitored frequently with dose titration until the chosen target urate concentration has been achieved. Once the target has been achieved, less frequent monitoring should continue to ensure that it is maintained. Management of acute flares necessitates rapid and effective control of the inflammatory response to monosodium urate crystals, thereby reducing joint pain and swelling. Guidelines recommend a non-steroidal anti-inflammatory drug (NSAID), colchicine, or corticosteroids. These drugs can be used alone or in combination for more severe flares. Gout flares may be precipitated by the introduction of intensive urate-lowering therapy and can continue to occur for many months after the target serum urate concentration has been achieved. Careful education about this possibility and the use of anti-inflammatories to prevent flares in the early phase of urate-lowering therapy is crucial, because such flares frequently result in poor adherence. Anti-inflammatory prophylaxis is recommended for at least 6 months from initiation of urate-lowering therapy. There are three main classes of medication to treat hyperuricemia. These are: medications that inhibit urate production (xanthine oxidase inhibitors), such as allopurinol and febuxostat; medications that normalize renal urate excretion (uricosurics), including probenecid, benzbromarone, and the newer novel urate transporter 1(URAT1) inhibitor lesinurad; and medications that catalyze the conversion of urate to the more water soluble and readily excretable allantoin (recombinant uricases), such as pegloticase and rasburicase.

REFERENCES

[1] March L, Smith RR, Woolf A et al. Burden of disability due to musculoskeletal (MSK) disorders. Best Practice and Research *Clinical Rheumatology* 2014; 28:353-366.

[2] Prince M, Wu F, Yusuf S et al. The burden of disease in older people and implications for health policy and practice. *Lancet* 2015; 385: 549-562.

[3] James SL, Abate D, Abate KH, et al. Global, regional and national incidence, prevalence and years lived with disability for 354 diseases and injuries for 195 countries and territories, 1990-2017: a systemic analysis for the Global Burden of disease study 2017. *Lancet* 2018; 392: 1789-858.

[4] Osteoarthritis: national clinical guideline for care and management in adults. In: Conditions. NCCfC (Ed), *Royal College of Physicians,* London 2008.

[5] Osteoarthritis research society international (OARSI). *Recommended performance based tests to assess physical function in people diagnosed with hip and knee osteoarthritis*. Available at: https://www.oarsi.org/sites/default/files/docs.

[6] Centers for disease control and prevention (CDC). *Osteoarthritis.* Available at: https://www.cdc.gov/arthritis/basics/osteoarthritis.htm. Accessed November 2020.

[7] World health Organization (WHO). *Chronic rheumatic conditions* Available at: http://www.who.int/chp/topics/rheumatic/en/. Accessed November 2020.

[8] *Oxford Textbook of Rheumatology* (4th Edition).

[9] Woolf A, Brooks P, Akesson K, Mody G. Prevention of musculoskeletal conditions in the developing world. *Best Practice & Research Clinical Rheumatology*. Vol 22, No 4, 759-772, 2008.

[10] Meuchi RD, Fassa AG, Faria NCX. Rev Saude Publica 2015; 49:1.

[11] Omokhodion, F. O., U. S. Umar, B. E. Ogunnowo. *Occupational Medicine*, Volume 50, Issue 2, February 2000, Pages 107–110.

[12] Will JS, Burn DC, Miller JA. *Am Fam Physician*. 2018 Oct 1; 98(7):421-428.

[13] Morris et al. *BMC Musculoskeletal Disorders* (2018) 19:196.

[14] Deyo RA, Rainville J, Kent DL. What can the history and physical examination tell us about low back pain? *JAMA*. 1992; 268 (6):760.

[15] Morris LD, Daniels KJ, Ganguli B and Louw QA. *BMC Musculoskeletal Disorders* 2018; 19:196.

[16] Hoy D., March L., Woolf A., Blyth F., Brooks P., Smith E. et al., 2014, 'The global burden of neck pain: Estimates from the global burden of disease 2010 study,' *Annals of Rheumatic Diseases* 73(7), 1309–1315.

[17] Hurwitz EL., Randhawa K., Yu H., Côté P. & Haldeman S., 2018, 'The global spine care initiative: A summary of the global burden of low back and neck pain studies,' *European Spine Journal* 27(Suppl 6), 796–801.

[18] Binder A. The diagnosis and treatment of nonspecific neck pain and whiplash. *Eura Medicophys* 2007; 43:79-89.

[19] Bester FCJ, Bosch FJ, and Jansen van Rensburg BJ. The specialist physician's approach to rheumatoid arthritis in South Africa. *Korean J Intern Med* 2016; 31: 219-23.

[20] Adelowo OO, Ojo O, Oduenyi I & Okwara CC. Rheumatoid arthritis among Nigerians: the first 200 patients from a rheumatology clinic. *Clinical Rheumatology* 2010; 29: 593-597.

[21] Smolen JS, Landewe R, Bijlsma J, Burmester G, Chatzidionysiou K, Dougados M, et al. EULAR recommendations for the management of rheumatoid arthritis with synthetic and biological disease-modifying anti- rheumatic drugs: 2016 update. *Ann Rheum Dis*. 2017; 76:960-977.

[22] Singh JA, Saag KG, Bridges SL Jr, Akl EA, Bannuru RR, Sullivan MC, et al. 2015 Ameri- can College of Rheumatology Guideline for the Treatment of Rheumatoid Arthritis. *Arthritis Rheumatol*. 2016; 68:1- 26.

[23] Lau CS, Chia F, Harrison A, Hsieh TY, Jain R, Jung SM, et al; Asia Pacific League of Associations for Rheumatology. APLAR

rheumatoid arthritis treatment recommendations. *Int J Rheum Dis.* 2015; 18:685-713.

[24] Dalbeth N, Merriman TR, Stamp LK. Gout. *Lancet* 2016; 388 (10055): 2039-2052.

[25] Ouedraogo DD, Lompo CP, Tieno H, Bognounou R, Diendere AE, Sawadogo A, et al. Rheumatic disorders observed in HIV infected patients undergoing highly active antiretroviral therapy (HAART): a 366-case prospective study in Burkina Faso. *Med Trop* (Mars). 2010; 70(4):345–8. Epub 2010/08/01.

[26] Genga EK, Oyoo GO, Kalla AA. The management of gout in Africa: challenges and opportunities. *Clinical Rheumatology* 2020 Sep 17.

[27] Fitzgerald et al. 2020 American College of Rheumatology guideline for the management of gout. *Arthritis care and Research*. 2020; 72: 6; 744-760.

In: Care of the Older African Adult
Editor: Seki A. Balogun
ISBN: 978-1-53619-295-7

Chapter 9

PAIN MANAGEMENT IN OLDER AFRICAN ADULTS

Akhtar Purvez*

Pain and Spine Center of Charlottesville, Charlottesville, VA, USA

ABSTRACT

Pain is a complex phenomenon that is affected by, and can in turn impact, many other conditions that are common in older adults - cognitive decline, mood changes, sleep, and low activity levels. A 2016 study found that 20% of adults in the United States experience chronic pain [1], a number that only increases with age. African adults experience low back pain at a rate higher than developed countries [2]. It is a leading cause of disability and greatly impacts quality of life. Common causes of chronic pain include degenerative joint and spine disease resulting in radicular and/or axial pain, myofascial pain and fibromyalgia, diabetic neuropathy, sickle cell disease, post-herpetic neuralgia and complex regional pain syndrome (CRPS). As the prevalence of diabetes is increasing in Africa and throughout the world [3], the number of those with the resulting complications including diabetic neuropathy will likely increase. In Africa, there is limited access to pain relieving medications, especially opioids, as well as interventional treatments that, in combination, are commonly utilized in the developed world. In addition, treatment may sometimes be

* Corresponding Author's Email: mansbal@yahoo.com.

limited to traditional healers in rural areas due to lack of access to medical care, which may lead to serious long-term complications as the diseases progress.

Keywords: Africans, African Americans, chronic pain, interventional pain management, older adults, opioid therapy, osteoarthritis, pain, postherpetic neuralgia, post-stroke pain syndrome, radiculopathy, sickle cell disease

1. Epidemiology of Pain in Africa

Older adults worldwide, regardless of ethnicity or race, experience pain. This is often related to degenerative joint and spine disease resulting in radicular and/or axial pain, myofascial pain, fibromyalgia, diabetic neuropathy, sickle cell disease, post-herpetic neuralgia, and complex regional pain syndrome (CRPS). There is limited information on how common these conditions are in Africa. A review of available studies on the prevalence of low back pain in Africa found that it is likely comparable to the rates in developed countries. On average, 50% of African adults experienced low back pain in the course of one year, while 62% experienced low back pain at some point in their lifetimes [4]. This is increasingly recognized as a major cause of disability; a Cameroon study of adults with low back pain found that 88% had a dysfunctional level of disability [5]. A study of Nigerian farmers found that load carrying on the head may be related to cervical spondylosis [6], emphasizing the need to examine occupational risk factors.

Sickle cell disease, a genetic illness that is more prevalent in people of African descent results in pain crises. The prevalence of the disease itself and the resulting sequelae, have increased over generations, mainly from improved survival of those with heterozygous sickle cell trait due to resistance to malaria, which is very common in many regions of sub-Saharan Africa. An estimated 240,000 children are born in sub-Saharan Africa with this disease [7]. Worldwide, there are 300,000 individuals with this ailment - a number that is projected to reach 400,000 by 2050 [8]. While this continues to be a common cause of childhood mortality in Africa, older individuals that survive will continue to experience chronic pain with recurrent acute exacerbations that require medical attention and frequent hospitalizations.

HIV/AIDs can result in peripheral neuropathy leading to chronic pain. There were an estimated 24.7 million individuals living with HIV in sub-Saharan Africa in 2014, which is 71% of the global population with HIV [9]. A systematic review revealed varying estimates of the prevalence of peripheral neuropathy in HIV patients, ranging from 1.2% to 69.4%. Older adults are more likely to develop HIV-related peripheral neuropathy and with greater severity [10].

2. Characteristics of Pain in Africa

Africa has low access to advanced medical expertise in many healthcare specialties including to chronic pain management. Access to opioids is often limited, even for palliative care for terminal conditions such as cancer or HIV/AIDS [11]. This is especially true for sub-Saharan Africa, though differences in availability of opioid therapy does vary throughout the region [12]. Only seven percent of health facilities in Kenya and Uganda were found to have morphine in a 2014 study [13]. Africa continues to have the lowest consumption of opioids of any continent, despite rising consumption worldwide [14]. A lack of pain research in Africa also limits our knowledge and may skew our understanding towards higher economic ranking countries such as Nigeria or South Africa [15].

3. Aging and the Development of Chronic Pain in Older Adults

Chronic pain is most common in older adults, increasing with age until age 65, where the rates remain stable for the rest of life. This is often related to the development of specific diseases associated with aging. Acute pain does not seem to vary with age [16].

3.1. Age Related Structural Changes

Like other body organs and systems, the spine and joints experience physiological changes with age. Normal aging process in combination with strain of everyday activities may result in the development or worsening of osteoarthritis involving the spine and major joints. People who are involved in activities that include heavy lifting, twisting, turning motions, or prolonged sitting or driving, are more prone to develop low back pain [17]. Issues with balance may result in falls that may cause injuries and lead to chronic pain. While older adults are less likely to sustain injuries at work, their injuries are likely to be more severe and result in long-lasting effects [18]. Spinal changes include dehydration of the intervertebral discs that are normally 60-80% water content, resulting in uneven pressure on the posterior column of the spinal cord and axial back pain; and to prolapse and displacement of discs, especially toward the posterior or posterior-lateral areas. This may result in spinal stenosis leading to compression of the spinal cord, foraminal stenosis and radiculopathy of the nerve distribution areas. Involvement of the hip joints and sacroiliac (SI) joints from osteoarthritis may also result in altered gait resulting in increased number of falls [19] and a vicious circle of physiological changes; as well as chronic pain. Similar changes may occur in other joints with aging, especially weight bearing joints such as knees and feet, subsequently resulting in chronic pain and decreased mobility. In addition, the risk of obesity in Africa and developed countries continues to impact bone health and leads to changes in weight bearing joints [20]. Because of obesity, they may also not be suitable candidates for reconstructive surgeries including joint replacement, creating a double loop of complications. Other chronic pain conditions including rheumatoid arthritis and gout are common and worsen with age.

4. Assessment of Pain in Older Adults

Pain is a complex phenomenon and as such, assessment requires attention to detail. Many older adults may have been experiencing pain for a decade or more, and therefore have tried a number of modalities. A comprehensive history will include discussing the location of the pain, the quality, duration, if it is constant or intermittent, and any instigating factors or injuries. A physical examination is then undertaken to figure out the extent and distribution of the pain and possible etiologies. Imaging, in the form of X-rays, CT and MRI may be required and are often helpful. Routinely, the level of the pain is measured from 0-10 by the Numeric Rating Scale (NRS 11). It may also be measured with other parameters including the Wong-Baker Faces Pain scale. These are subjective measures that allow for patients to express how much pain they are experiencing. Cultural differences may inform the way patients perceive and communicate about their pain. Africa has many heterogeneous cultures that may vary in their beliefs surrounding pain. Nortje et al. conducted interviews from individuals of various South African cultures and a report of the results follow. In the Nguni culture, beliefs around pain are centered on communication with ancestors while in the Sotho culture, there is the belief that pain is punishment from angered spirits called Balimo [21]. These beliefs may discourage such individuals from speaking out about pain and influence the types of treatment, patients are willing to seek out. A traditional healer may have been the first line of treatment, either out of necessity because there is no access to Western medicine, or because traditional medicine is preferred. Interviews conducted also revealed that men are not expected to reveal pain, while women are expected to speak up or cry out to show they are in physical pain. Health care providers (HCPs) should be aware of any cultural or personal beliefs that may affect how the patient displays or speaks about pain. Assessment of pain requires understanding and the development of a strong relationship with the HCPs and formulating a treatment plan that aligns with the patients' beliefs and values. A history of previous treatments, including pharmacologic, physical therapy, interventional procedures or injections, can be useful in determining a course of action. Patients that have tried many of these treatments without success may be candidates for a surgical consult or other referral. Cognitive decline or impairment in older adults may impede discussing pain and the ability of the patient to communicate the level and areas of pain. Caregivers and family members may be important to create a clearer picture of the pain and the patient's history and to ensure compliance with the proposed management plan. A remarkable study reported on a geriatrician-led house call program because home-based medical care is increasingly being utilized in many developed and developing countries. This is crucial for many frail older adults with significant functional and/or cognitive issues [22].

5. Common Conditions Resulting in Chronic Pain in Older Africa Adults

There is a varied group of conditions that may result in chronic pain in this population group as discussed above. A wider review of some of the more common conditions follows.

5.1. Myofascial and Skeletal Pain

Older adults often present with joint or back pain related to osteoarthritis, and many may believe it to be a natural or normal result of aging that they must live with. Details on osteoarthritis are presented in the chapter on "Musculoskeletal Diseases in Older Adults" and this chapter will focus on the resultant pain and its management. Aging does result in degenerative processes such as osteoarthritis and degenerative disc disease, which can result in pain and disability. This can limit mobility, activities of daily living, and reduce quality of life among older adults. It is important to determine the effect the pain is having on their day-to-day life, which may also involve speaking to caregivers or family members. Pain of the lumbar and cervical spine is most common. This type of pain is usually accompanied by muscle spasm, stiffness and sometimes gait changes that may further limit their functional quality of life. The first line of treatment usually include acetaminophen, NSAIDs, stretching and movement, rest, heat, and ice. For medication management in older adults, the Beers Criteria for inappropriate medication use in older patients should be consulted when deciding to prescribe a medication [23]. NSAIDs may be contraindicated in older adults due to other illnesses or medications, and should be avoided for long term, daily, continuous use due to risks including those of renal damage. Also, adults that are taking low-dose aspirin to prevent heart attack or stroke should not take NSAIDs due to an interaction that may reduce the therapeutic efficacy of aspirin. To reduce these risks, Cox 2 inhibitors like celecoxib is an option but the risks of gastrointestinal bleeding must still be considered when prescribing these medications. Topical medications such as lidocaine or diclofenac may be a reasonable option to reduce systemic absorption. Various classes of muscle relaxant medications including baclofen, cyclobenzaprine, metaxalone or tizanidine can also provide relief of associated reflex spasm that is usually part of the symptom complex. However, many of these latter medications may result in sedation and dizziness. The patients, and their caregivers should be warned about this and closely monitored to avoid potential falls that may result in injury. Polypharmacy is common in older adults. It is estimated that at least 30% of older adults are taking five or more medications [24]. People in advanced ages may be taking medications for hypertension, diabetes mellitus, high cholesterol, hypothyroidism or for other medical issues. The risks of drug-drug interactions and resulting serious complications should be considered, addressed and patients monitored closely. It may be necessary to consult with their primary care physician before prescribing any medications. In many situations, it may be appropriate to keep all medications “under one roof” and preferably prescribed by the primary care physician to reduce these risks.

In some parts of Africa, medicinal plants and traditional healing is the most accessible and affordable way to receive treatment [25]. Some of the traditional medicines and substance used may have medicinal properties and some genuine therapeutic effects including anti-inflammatory effects as seen with NSAIDS. A study of extracts of medicinal plants used for pain relief in Africa found that many of them had high COX-1 or COX-2 inhibitory activity [26]. There is a large diversity of these medicinal plants, and not all of them have been studied. In a clinical setting, there may be concerns about risks including toxicity with these plants and other remedies that have not been studied or regulated. As such, and because the ingredients and formulation of these medications cannot be controlled, these should be avoided, particularly in older adults.

Physical therapy can provide significant relief in many ailments and should be part of most of the management plans. If this is not possible, a home exercise plan involving regular walking, yoga, or other stretching and exercise programs should be discussed. This would be beneficial generally for the overall health of patients and specifically to reduce chronic pain and risks of further injury by core building, strengthening and improving the range of motion.

In addition to physical therapy, a comprehensive management plan may include medications and interventional pain management approaches. In majority of patients, these, in combination are able to keep their symptoms under control and keep them functional. Surgery, if indicated, is usually considered the last option. Many patients with myofascial pain may benefit from trigger point injections into the muscles, usually containing a local anesthetic and/or steroid. These are minimally invasive and can relieve muscle spasms temporarily, allowing for increased movement and participation in a physical therapy or exercise program. Intra-articular corticosteroid injections for the shoulder, hip or knee joint may also improve pain symptoms in these joints, if osteoarthritis is confirmed by imaging.

There are several interventional procedure options for back pain resulting from osteoarthritis of the spine and joints. Imaging including X-rays followed by CT, MRI or bone scans of the spine may reveal degenerative joint and disc disease and spondylosis, including facet arthropathy, spinal and foraminal stenosis. There may also be osteoarthritis of the hips or the sacroiliac joints, in which case steroid injections of these areas under fluoroscopic guidance may be performed. If the patient describes pain that is mostly axial and that does not radiate down extremities, it may be appropriate to perform diagnostic medial branch blocks of the affected areas. If this results in temporary relief, even for a brief period of time, this is followed up with radiofrequency ablation, or denervation, which can provide relief for 3-6 months, and sometimes longer. These procedures can be repeated at intervals, if needed.

Knee pain that is not responsive to physical therapy, NSAIDs, intermittent steroid injections, may be responsive to genicular nerve blocks. This may be followed by genicular nerve ablation that usually result in relief lasting several months. Patients that are not candidates for joint replacement may also be a candidate for novel approaches, including peripheral nerve stimulation (PNS) of infrapatellar saphenous nerves. Similarly, patients with back pain that continues to be unresponsive to extensive conservative management or spinal surgery may be a candidate for spinal or peripheral nerve stimulation. Axial low back and hip area pain in some cases may be a result of involvement of the cluneal nerves. This an often a missed and underdiagnosed condition that is empirically responsive to a PNS approach in many patients.

5.2. Neuropathic Pain and Central Pain

This type of pain is characterized by burning, numbness or tingling described by the patient. This may result from multiple etiologies including diabetic peripheral neuropathy, postherpetic neuralgia, nerve compression syndromes, complex regional pain syndrome (CRPS) and strokes. There are multiple pharmacological options that target neuropathy. Medications including antiepileptic drugs like gabapentin and pregabalin and serotonin norepinephrine reuptake inhibitors like duloxetine may be considered and are very effective in many patients, though dosages may need to be gradually titrated and optimized to a therapeutic level. This approach allows for time for patients to get acclimatized to the drugs and to watch for side effects including sedation and balance issues. Some patients may need higher dosages of one of these medications or a combination of medications to increase the symbiotic effect and try to keep the risks of toxicity low. These should also be tapered down slowly, if required, to avoid withdrawal effects including seizures. Patients that need to discontinue these medications may need to be provided with a written schedule to follow.

The pain that radiates down from spine to an extremity is considered radicular and is likely resulting from neural foraminal or spinal stenosis. Frequently, this is a result of age-related degenerative spinal changes. Conservative management such as physical therapy, NSAIDS, anti-neuropathic medications described above as well as epidural steroid injections are the preferred treatment for radiculopathy. A surgical consult with a neurosurgeon or orthopedic surgeon should be discussed if the symptoms do not improve or worsen. Progression to severe neurological situations including weakness and bladder or bowel issues demand urgent consultation and possible surgery. Decompressive surgery usually accompanied by fusion carries a longer recovery period and increased risks for older adults. Unfortunately, some of these patients may either not improve or see recurrence of symptoms within a few years of the initial surgery necessitating additional surgeries.

Neuropathic pain in older adults is also commonly caused by diabetes mellitus. High blood sugar levels damage the nerves and lead to peripheral neuropathy, usually in the typical 'glove and stocking' pattern. HIV infection may result in many serious complications chronically including peripheral neuropathy. This may also occur from some antiretroviral therapy used to treat this infection. Trials on therapeutic medications have shown limited success and most medications traditionally used for neuropathy have not provided more relief than placebos in those with HIV neuropathy. Capsaicin, smoked cannabis, and recombinant human nerve growth factor have shown greater pain relief than the placebo [27]. In spite of these assertions, the traditional anti-neuropathic medications described elsewhere in this chapter should be tried and may offer significant relief in some patients.

Postherpetic neuralgia occurs almost exclusively in older adults. Many individuals with shingles recover completely, but a small proportion continue to have excruciating pain usually involving one or more dermatomes on the same side that stops at the midline. A prophylactic shingles vaccine is recommended in older adults. This is generally a series of two vaccines that usually results in many years of protection. If a shingles rash occurs, the patient should receive antiviral medication which is more effective if started very early in the course of the disease. In the long-term anti-neuropathic medications, topical analgesia and, in resistant cases, peripheral nerve or spinal stimulation may be tried.

Following a cerebrovascular accident, some patients develop central post-stroke pain syndrome (CPSP), usually involving neuropathic pain on one side of the body. These patients may be difficult to manage but the general approach of employing anti-neuropathic drugs does provide significant relief for many of these patients, if they tolerate these medications. These medications mainly include anti-depressants like duloxetine and anti-seizure drugs like gabapentin and pregabalin. Patients may also have musculoskeletal pain or pain associated with spasticity or shoulder subluxation [28]. Since hypertension, a risk factor for stroke, is more prevalent in people of African descent [29], strokes and subsequent pain syndromes logically, may also be more frequent.

5.3. Sickle Cell Disease

Sickle cell disease is often fatal in Africa and is a common cause of premature death. These consequences are thought to be mainly due to infectious diseases and bacterial infections. Those that survive describe episodes of acute pain, as well as ongoing chronic pain, as one of the most difficult aspects of managing this disease. Acute pain episodes are thought to be caused by vaso-occlusion and while it does not appear to cause organ damage, it results in emergency room visits and decreased quality of life [30]. While the mechanisms are still not completely understood, it may be related to vaso-occlusion and sickling and from dehydration.

The American Society of Hematology's (ASH) 2020 guidelines for sickle cell disease recommend an interdisciplinary approach involving the individual's entire care team for the management of pain. The main treatment for acute pain is opioids in addition to managing other associated conditions like dehydration. An individualized care plan is recommended by the ASH, which includes treatments and dosages that have been effective in the past. ASH also recommends a 5 to 7 day course of NSAIDs alongside opioid therapy. Sickle cell patients may have other comorbidities related to involvement of kidneys or other organs, so NSAID usage should be personalized and considered in the wider context of the patient's health. Other recommendations include ketamine infusion, regional anesthesia, TENS, massage, or yoga [31].

Unfortunately, other modalities of treatment such as corticosteroids, either to relieve pain or shorten the episode of pain, have not proved effective (30). Chronic pain in individuals with sickle cell disease may also be caused by avascular necrosis of bone, or have no known distinct etiology. For patients with necrosis of bone, SNRIs and NSAIDs are recommended. For those with no known cause, SNRIs, gabapentinoids (gabapentin, pregabalin), tricyclic antidepressants, and cognitive/ behavioral strategies are recommended [31]. As life expectancy for individuals with sickle cell increases, it will become more common in older adults. The treatment for acute pain crises does not change with age, though there may be concerns about prescribing opioids for older adults because of possible adverse effects.

5.4. Fibromyalgia

Fibromyalgia is characterized by chronic widespread myofascial pain, usually accompanied by fatigue, memory issues, and sleep/mood disturbances. It is sometimes referred to as "centralized pain", since it originates or is amplified by the central nervous system. If imaging and physical examination do not reveal an underlying cause for pain, fibromyalgia should be considered. The main treatment is exercise and cognitive behavioral therapy, as well as tricyclic antidepressants, SNRIs, and gabapentinoids [32]. There are three specifically approved medications for this condition including duloxetine, milnacipran and pregabalin.

6. Emerging Treatments for Chronic Pain

Cannabidiol (CBD) oil, cannabis, and Tetrahydrocannabinol (THC) extracts are increasingly popular for chronic pain. The legality by state and country varies for these substances. In some states/countries, patients may not be willing to disclose this information. In other areas, providers may be able to provide a marijuana card for patients with chronic pain. Kratom, *Mitragyna speciosa*, is also a popular plant extract that contains agonists for opioid receptors and is used by some individuals for chronic pain or opioid withdrawal [33]. However, there are reports of toxicity and adverse effects, as well as addiction. In general, the health care providers are best served staying with the accepted standard of care; and using approved, well researched medications and non-pharmacological approaches.

7. Opioid Therapy in Older Adults

Opioid therapy for chronic pain is controversial due to potential risks, especially in older patients. Benzodiazepines in combination with opioids can result in severe respiratory depression and death. Older adults with other conditions, such as sleep apnea, are not good candidates. With a multitude of other available medications, opioids should not be considered as first line of management. Trials with non-opioid therapies should be attempted first. A small dose of opioids such as oxycodone, hydrocodone, or tramadol can be helpful for breakthrough pain for certain patients. However, this requires careful observation, discussion about risks, and monitoring for adverse effects [34].

8. Adults of African Descent in the United States of America

Adults of African descent in America are considered by the medical field to be Black/African American, a diverse group that cannot be generalized. Recent immigrants from Africa or their children may have unique cultural backgrounds as well as genetic histories. Many will face many of the biases that African Americans do today. Black Americans are less likely to be prescribed opioids or receive pain management treatment than white Americans [35]. This disparity can be attributed in part to racial bias, as found by a 2016 study of medical students. These students were found to have false beliefs, including that Black people may have thicker skin [36]. Clinicians should consider their own implicit biases; and the training and education of residents and fellows should be stressed to make them aware of these issues.

References

[1] Dahlhamer J, Lucas J, Zelaya, C, et al. Prevalence of Chronic Pain and High-Impact Chronic Pain among Adults — United States, 2016. *MMWR Morb. Mortal Wkly Rep.* 2018; 67:1001–1006.

[2] Morris L D, Daniels K J, Ganguli B, Louw Q A. An update on the prevalence of low back pain in Africa: a systematic review and meta-analyses. *BMC Musculoskelet. Disord.* 2018; 19(1):196. Published 2018 Jun 21.

[3] Mbanya J C, Ramiaya K. Diabetes Mellitus. In: Jamison DT, Feachem R G, Makgoba M W, et al., editors. *Disease and Mortality in Sub-Saharan Africa.* 2nd edition. Washington (DC): The International Bank for Reconstruction and Development / The World Bank; 2006. Chapter 19.

[4] Louw Q A, Morris LD, Grimmer-Somers K. The prevalence of low back pain in Africa: a systematic review. *BMC Musculoskelet. Disord.* 2007 Nov 1; 8:105.

[5] Doualla M, Aminde J, Aminde L N, Lekpa F K, Kwedi F M, Yenshu E V, Chichom A M. Factors influencing disability in patients with chronic low back pain attending a tertiary hospital in sub-Saharan Africa. *BMC Musculoskelet. Disord.* 2019 Jan 15; 20(1):25.

[6] Oguntona S A. Cervical spondylosis in South West Nigerian farmers and female traders. *Ann. Afr. Med.* 2014 Apr-Jun; 13(2):61-4.

[7] Williams T N. Sickle Cell Disease in Sub-Saharan Africa. *Hematol. Oncol. Clin. North Am.* 2016 Apr; 30(2):343-58.

[8] Piel F B, Hay S I, Gupta S, Weatherall DJ, Williams TN. Global burden of sickle cell anaemia in children under five, 2010-2050: modelling based on demographics, excess mortality, and interventions. *PLoS Med.* 2013; 10(7).

[9] Joint United Nations Programme on HIV/AIDS (UNAIDS). *The Gap Report*. 2014.

[10] Ghosh S, Chandran A, Jansen J P. Epidemiology of HIV-related neuropathy: a systematic literature review. *AIDS Res. Hum. Retroviruses.* 2012 Jan; 28(1):36-48.

[11] Harding R, Profrene J, Higginson I J. Palliative care in sub-Saharan Africa. *Lancet.* 2005; 365:1971–7.

[12] Nchako E, Bussell S, Nesbeth C, Odoh C. Barriers to the availability and accessibility of controlled medicines for chronic pain in Africa. *Int. Health.* 2018 Mar 1; 10(2):71-77.

[13] Harding R, Simms V, Penfold S, Downing J, Powell R A, Mwangi-Powell F, Namisango E, Moreland S, Gikaara N, Atieno M, Kataike J, Nsubuga C, Munene G, Banga G, Higginson I J. Availability of essential drugs for managing HIV-related pain and symptoms within 120 PEPFAR-funded health facilities in East Africa: a cross-sectional survey with onsite verification. *Palliat. Med.* 2014 Apr; 28(4):293-301.

[14] International Narcotics Control Board. *Progress in Ensuring Adequate Access to Internationally Controlled Substances for Medical and Scientific Purposes*. 2019. doi: 10.18356/9b973caa-en.

[15] Onyeka T C, Chukwuneke F N. Pain research in Africa: a ten-year bibliometric survey. *J. Anesth.* 2014 Aug; 28(4):511-6.

[16] Bicket M C, Mao J. Chronic Pain in Older Adults. *Anesthesiol. Clin.* 2015 Sep; 33(3):577-90.

[17] Pope, Malcolm H.; Goh, Kheng Lim; Magnusson, Marianne L. *Annual Review of Biomedical Engineering*. 2002, Vol. 4 Issue 1, p49.

[18] Stoesz B, Chimney K, Deng C, et al. Incidence, risk factors, and outcomes of non-fatal work-related injuries among older workers: A review of research from 2010 to 2019. *Safety Science.* 2020; 126: N.PAG.

[19] Smith T O, Higson E, Pearson M, Mansfield M. Is there an increased risk of falls and fractures in people with early diagnosed hip and knee osteoarthritis? Data from the Osteoarthritis Initiative. *International Journal of Rheumatic Diseases.* 2018; 21(6):1193-1201.

[20] King L K, March L, Anandacoomarasamy A. Obesity & osteoarthritis. *Indian Journal of Medical Research.* 2013; 138(2):185-193.

[21] Nortjé, N, Albertyn R. The cultural language of pain: a South African study. *South African Family Practice.* 2015; 57(1): 24-27.

[22] Balogun, S A, Osi-Ogbu, O. Geriatric House Calls: A Geriatrician-Led Clinical Experience in Sub-Saharan *Africa. Gerontol Geratr. Res.* 2020; 1(1): 4-4.

[23] By the 2019 American Geriatrics Society Beers Criteria® Update Expert Panel. American Geriatrics Society 2019 Updated AGS Beers Criteria® for Potentially Inappropriate Medication Use in Older Adults. *J. Am. Geriatr. Soc*. 2019 Apr; 67(4):674-694.

[24] Qato D M, Wilder J, Schumm L P, Gillet V, Alexander G C. Changes in Prescription and Over-the-Counter Medication and Dietary Supplement Use among Older Adults in the United States, 2005 vs 2011. *JAMA Intern. Med.* 2016 Apr; 176(4):473-82.

[25] Oguntibeju O O. Medicinal plants with anti-inflammatory activities from selected countries and regions of Africa. *J. Inflamm. Res*. 2018 Aug 7; 11:307-317.

[26] Fawole O A, Amoo S O, Ndhlala A R, Light M E, Finnie J F, Van Staden J. Anti-inflammatory, anticholinesterase, antioxidant and phytochemical properties of medicinal plants used for pain-related ailments in South Africa. *Journal of Ethnopharmacology.* 2010; 127 (2):235-241.

[27] Kaku M, Simpson D M. HIV neuropathy. *Curr. Opin. HIV AIDS.* 2014 Nov; 9(6):521-6.

[28] Harrison R A, Field T S. Post stroke pain: identification, assessment, and therapy. *Cerebrovasc. Dis.* 2015; 39(3-4):190-201.

[29] Yoon S S, Carroll M D, Fryar C D. Hypertension Prevalence and Control among Adults: United States, 2011-2014. *NCHS Data Brief.* 2015 Nov; (220):1-8.

[30] Rees D C, Williams T N, Gladwin M T. Sickle-cell disease. *Lancet.* 2010 Dec 11; 376(9757):2018-31.

[31] Brandow A M, Carroll C P, Creary S, et al. American Society of Hematology 2020 guidelines for sickle cell disease: management of acute and chronic pain. *Blood Adv.* 2020; 4(12):2656-2701.

[32] Clauw D J. Fibromyalgia: A Clinical Review. *JAMA*. 2014; 311(15): 1547–1555.

[33] Ismail I, Wahab S, Sidi H, Das S, Lin L J, Razali R. Kratom and Future Treatment for the Opioid Addiction and Chronic Pain: Periculo Beneficium? *Curr. Drug. Targets*. 2019; 20(2):166-172.

[34] Purvez A. *Managing Chronic Pain in an Age of Addiction.* Lanham, Maryland: Rowman & Littlefield; 2018.

[35] Campbell C M, Edwards R R. Ethnic differences in pain and pain management. *Pain Manag*. 2012; 2(3):219-230.

[36] Hoffman K M, Trawalter S, Axt J R, Oliver M N. Racial bias in pain assessment and treatment recommendations, and false beliefs about biological differences between blacks and whites. *Proc. Natl. Acad. Sci. U S A*. 2016; 113(16):4296-4301.

In: Care of the Older African Adult
Editor: Seki A. Balogun
ISBN: 978-1-53619-295-7

Chapter 10

ENDOCRINE DISORDERS IN OLDER ADULTS OF AFRICAN DESCENT

***Oluyemisi Abdulsalam*[1,*] *and Omolola Olajide*[2,†]**
[1]Clinical Endocrinologist, Veterans Affairs Medical Center, Fayetteville, NC, US
[2]Associate Professor, Internal Medicine, Section of Endocrinology Marshall School of Medicine, Huntington, WV, US

ABSTRACT

Endocrine disorders fall into broad categories of hormone over and underproduction, altered tissue response to hormones or tumors arising from endocrine tissue with equally wide degree of clinical characteristics in older Africans. Prevalence, clinical manifestations and management of these disorders vary widely depending on the actual disease entity. Diabetes Mellitus is the most common endocrinopathy with incidence increasing with age and obesity. In general, older individuals tend to lead a more sedentary lifestyle. Obesity is sometimes viewed as a sign of affluence and not a risk factor for disease in the African culture. In

* Corresponding Author's Email: oluyemisi.abdulsalam@va.gov.
† Corresponding Author's Email: Olajideo@marshall.edu.

particular, individuals of African descent tend to have diets high in carbohydrates. This, coupled with less physical activity, can lead to glucose intolerance and subsequent progression to overt diabetes. The second most common endocrinology disorders are thyroid disorders which include hypothyroidism, hyperthyroidism, thyroid nodules/goiters and thyroid cancer. Endocrine disorders are sometimes diagnosed late in the course of the disease for various reasons such as lack of access to care, low socio-economic status, genetic and regional or environmental factors. Other less common endocrinopathies worthy of mention in the older African population include disorders of bone and mineral metabolism such as osteoporosis, parathyroid disorders, pituitary abnormalities and adrenal disorders.

In this chapter, we review the most common endocrine disorders in older individuals of African descent, their unique clinical characteristics, complications and management, effects of poverty and lack of access to care on the disease burden in this geographic region.

Keywords: type 1 diabetes mellitus, type 2 diabetes mellitus, impaired fasting glucose, impaired glucose tolerance, pre-diabetes, diabetes ketoacidosis, hyperosmolar hyperglycemic nonketotic state, hypothyroidism, hyperthyroidism, graves' disease, Toxic Multinodular goiter (TMNG), fine needle aspiration, thyroid nodules, thyroid cancer, bone mineral density, FRAX score, dual energy x-ray absorptiometry, osteoporosis, osteopenia, fractures, hypoparathyroidism, primary hyperparathyroidism, secondary hyperparathyroidism, parathyroid cancer

1. Diabetes Mellitus

Diabetes Mellitus (DM) is a disease characterized by elevated plasma glucose. Most common types of diabetes mellitus include the following: pre-diabetes, type 1 diabetes mellitus (T1DM), type 2 diabetes mellitus (T2DM). Other types of diabetes include maturity onset diabetes of the young (MODY), latent autoimmune diabetes of adult (LADA) and ketosis prone diabetes (KPD). Prediabetes is highly prevalent in older persons. The diagnostic criteria are: impaired fasting glucose (IFG) with a fasting plasma glucose (FPG) of 100-125, impaired glucose tolerance (IGT) with 2-hour post prandial blood glucose (2HPPBG) of 140-199 or hemoglobin A1c (HbA1c) of 6-6.4%. An oral glucose tolerance test (OGTT) may be indicated as an additional test to make a diagnosis in older adults. Importantly, individuals with prediabetes are at increased risk for progression to diabetes and development of cardiovascular disease (CVD). Positive health interventions such as health education and counseling, healthy eating habits, exercise, access to healthcare are proven to be highly effective in delaying progression of prediabetes to overt diabetes mellitus in all age groups.

TIDM is characterized by relative or absolute lack of insulin often caused by autoimmune destruction of beta islet cells in the pancreas. This is often diagnosed in children and young adults but can also present for the first time in older individuals.

T2DM is characterized by insulin resistance, relative lack of insulin or both, as underlying pathophysiology. This accounts for over 90% of diabetes in adults with prevalence increasing with age. Risk factors include older age, obesity, hypertension, family history, metabolic syndrome, existence of prediabetes. Most of the discussion in this section will relate to T2DM.

With LADA, patients have features present in both T1DM and T2DM with measurable antibodies and presence of environmental risk factors similar to T2DM such as older age of onset, obesity, sedentary lifestyle, physical inactivity and smoking [1].

KPD is a common presentation of newly diagnosed individuals of African descent with type 2 diabetes. This has been previously referred to as Flatbush Diabetes, type 1.5 diabetes or atypical diabetes. This has also been described to a lesser extent in other minority non-European populations across the globe [2]. Patients with KPD often present acutely with diabetes ketoacidosis (DKA) without typical phenotypic appearance of T1DM, rather they are similar to T2DM in physical appearance. Various subgroups exist and are classified based on antibody status and beta islet cell reserve which can determine how quickly these patients can get off insulin or all antidiabetic medications. In some instances, this may be shortly after the acute DKA episode is treated. MODY will not be discussed in this chapter given its often diagnosed in young individuals before age 25.

1.1. Epidemiology

In 2019, the International Diabetes Federation (IDF) Atlas reported a global estimate of 9.3% of all adults aged 20 -79 years are living with DM which is equivalent to about 463 million people; and about 24% of these are 65 years and older. By 2030, the global prevalence of diabetes is projected to be up to 578 million adults with a third being 65 years and older and by 2045, this will be even higher at 700 million adults with almost 40% being 65 years and older. Africa has one of the lowest age adjusted prevalence of DM of about 4.7% with projections of up to 5.2% in 2045. It is estimated that about half of individuals with DM are not aware of their diagnosis hence risk of disease progression and complications remains high. Globally, 11.3% deaths are due to diabetes with at least half occurring in individuals age 60 years and older [3]. This is concerning given the progressive aging of populations worldwide. According to the 2019 United Nations report, one in eleven people worldwide were 65 years and older, which is projected to increase to one in six by 2050. The fastest growth is in North Africa and Western Asia, where there is a projected increase in the older adult population of over 220% and in sub-Saharan Africa (SSA), there is a projected growth of over 200% [4]. In the United States, the prevalence of diagnosed T1DM and T2DM are 0.5% and 8.5% respectively in adults, with T2DM making up about 91% of all cases and T1DM in only 5.6% [5]. The highest rates of increased DM prevalence are predominately in older adults and racial minorities [6]. In most African countries and in people of African descent worldwide, there are no consistent data on the incidence and prevalence of diabetes. Few publications with varying methodologies suggest prevalence of 9.2%, 5.8%, 2.4%, 1.4% in South Africa, Nigeria, Kenya and Uganda respectively [7-9]. DM is also associated with poorer quality of life scores and greater disability in these countries [7]. In particular, diabetes awareness is very low in SSA, with levels of awareness between 35–51% [8]. Identifying the true scope of the disease burden associated with DM in these countries, is very important, given the significant ongoing economic and governmental challenges. This is generally more difficult in underdeveloped countries with inadequate resources.

1.2. Clinical Diagnosis and Management

Older adults are typically diagnosed during routine laboratory screening or may present with symptoms of hyperglycemia. These symptoms include increased frequency of urination, polyuria, increased thirst (polydipsia), unintentional weight loss despite hyperphagia, blurry vision, tiredness, fatigue or generalized weakness. The diagnostic laboratory criteria include one or more of the following: FPG of 126mg/dl and above, 2HPPBG of 200mg/dl and above, HbA1c 6.5% and above. Diabetes mellitus may be diagnosed with any of above laboratory findings in the presence of hyperglycemic symptoms OR any of above laboratory criteria confirmed on 2 occasions without the presence of hyperglycemic symptoms. It is recommended to avoid using HbA1c as single diagnostic criteria for making initial diagnosis in older individuals over 65 years, especially blacks, and individuals with conditions that can affect hemoglobin levels such as hemoglobinopathies, hemolytic anemias, thalassemias, iron deficiency, severe hepatic or renal disease, spherocytosis, which are common in populations of African descent. In older individuals, it is also recommended to perform a 2-hr OGTT for confirmation of the diagnosis when suspected by fasting plasma glucose or HbA1c criteria [10]. In suspected cases of T1DM, other necessary labs that could help clinch diagnosis and make a distinction between T1DM and T2DM include c-peptide level, presence of relevant antibodies such as anti GAD65 antibody and islet cell antibody. It is important to note that these antibodies are not detectable in every type 1 diabetic. Patients with LADA have features present in both T1DM and T2DM with measurable antibodies and presence of environmental risk factors similar to T2DM such as older age of onset, obesity, sedentary lifestyle, physical inactivity and smoking [11]. Patients with KPD may also have presence or absence of antibodies. Older patients may also present with acute diabetic complications including: DKA, characterized by hyperglycemia symptoms described above in setting of acute metabolic acidosis, multiple electrolyte disturbances and possibly coma. This is most often seen in T1DM but can also occur in T2DM or Ketosis Prone Diabetics. In hyperglycemic hyperosmolar non-ketotic (HHNK) state, patients present with hyperosmolar state as a result of severe hyperglycemia, other electrolyte derangement, and possible coma, but with little or no acidosis.

The treatment of DM mainly involves lifestyle modification and pharmacotherapy. Great emphasis is placed on lifestyle management and weight loss for overweight or obese individuals. As little as 5% weight loss can be beneficial in lowering overall cardiovascular risk. Dietary recommendations include small to medium portion sized meals, high fiber, high protein, low carbohydrates and reduction or elimination of high intake of simple sugars. Exercise recommendations aim for minimum 150 minutes of exercise weekly in divided sessions, at least 30 mins/day, and five days/week. Patients are generally advised to gradually advance and maintain these goals as tolerated. Avoidance of smoking and other forms of tobacco use is also recommended, as well as adequate control of other modifiable cardiovascular risk factors such as hypertension, hyperlipidemia and obesity. Glucose monitoring is an integral part of DM management. This can be achieved by fingerstick blood glucose (FSBG) monitoring using a glucometer or continuous glucose monitoring systems (CGM).

Pharmacotherapy in T1DM largely involves insulin. Most of the antidiabetic medications discussed in this section are for treatment of T2DM. Any antidiabetic medication considered should be in combination with lifestyle management efforts. In older individuals, treatment goals and targets should depend on several factors including age, functional and cognitive ability in addition to presence of other comorbidities [10]. Other factors that should be considered include risk of hypoglycemia, simplicity of medication regimen, access to care, cost of medications and life expectancy. In older individuals residing in residential facilities with multiple caregivers, clear glucose targets should be established with emphasis on avoidance of hypoglycemia. All treatments decisions should be a shared decision making effort between the clinical provider, patient and care givers where applicable, to improve chances of compliance, treatment success and re-adjustment based on treatment success. Medications should be started if lifestyle management alone is not enough to achieve glycemic control or if based on set targets, patients will require more than lifestyle management alone at onset of disease.

The classes of antidiabetic medications are:

1.2.1.1. Biguanides

The mode of action (MoA) is to increase muscle glucose uptake and hepatic gluconeogenesis. Metformin is the most commonly available medication in this group and is the first line medication option for T2DM. In older individuals with chronic kidney disease, metformin may be contraindicated or dose adjustments necessary based on the stage of chronic kidney disease (CKD). This also applies to some other antidiabetic medications whose metabolism can be affected by varying stages of reduction in kidney function. It is recommended to avoid use in patients with heart failure or stage 4 CKD to avoid increased risk of lactic acidosis.

1.2.1.2. Sulphonylureas (SU)

Act to increase insulin production from pancreatic islet cells. First generation SU such as chlorpropramide, tolazamide, tolbutamide and acetohexamide (which is no longer in use), have largely been replaced by second generation options in most part of the world but are still in use in some countries. The second generation SU are glibenclamide, glimepiride, glipizide and gliclazide. These are more efficacious than first generation SU and can be used in lower doses. Major side effect of these medications is hypoglycemia with increased risk in older populations with or without kidney disease.

1.2.1.3. Glucagon-Like Peptide (GLP)-1 Agonist Therapies

This class of medications has been available since 2005. They act to directly increase meal related insulin production and decrease in glucagon secretion in a glucose dependent fashion, as well indirectly increase early satiety by slowing gastric emptying. The overall reduction in food intake often results in limiting weight gain or outright weight loss. Currently available preparations include liraglutide, semaglutide, dulaglutide and lixisenatide. The side effects of this class of medications include gastro-intestinal intolerance with nausea, vomiting, abdominal discomfort, pancreatitis and mild increased risk of medullary thyroid cancer. It is recommended that they be avoided in individuals who have had bariatric or bowel resection surgery or have gastroparesis. These medications can also cause hypoglycemia when used in conjunction with SU and insulin hence dose adjustments may be indicated. They are very effective when used as monotherapies or in conjunction with metformin, insulin or other antidiabetic class of drugs except DPP 4 inhibitors

1.2.1.4. Dipeptidyl Peptidase (DPP) 4 Inhibitors

This class of medications act to inhibit breakdown of naturally occurring incretins hence prolonging their duration of action in improving glucose dependent insulin release from pancreatic islet cells, decreasing meal dependent glucagon release and reducing gastric emptying. Though similar in action, they are not as potent or efficacious as GLP 1 agonist medications. Currently available preparations include sitagliptin, saxagliptin, linagliptin, alogliptin and vildagliptin which is only available outside the US. With the exception of linagliptin, most of these may need renal dose adjustments, especially with older populations. Pancreatitis remains a possible side effect, as well as increased risk of heart failure decompensation, in particular with saxagliptin and alogliptin. It is still unclear if this is a class effect.

1.2.1.5. Sodium Glucose Cotransporter (SGLT) 2 Inhibitors

These act to selectively inhibit the SGLT 2 proteins in the proximal renal tubule (which is responsible for about 90% of filtered glucose reabsorption), thereby reducing the renal threshold for glycosuria resulting in increased glycosuria and lowering of plasma glucose. None of its actions is via the pancreas hence these medications can be used irrespective of duration of T2DM as long as there is no significant renal failure. Currently available types are canagliflozin, dapagliflozin, empagliflozin and ertugliflozin. Other brands available outside the United States include ipragliflozin, tofogliflozin. These medications can be used as monotherapies or in combination with other antidiabetic drug medications. Other benefits that have been found with SGLT-2 inhibitors include weight loss, cardiovascular benefits (such as lower blood pressure, lower heart failure incidence, hospitalization and lowering of cardiovascular mortality) and renoprotection (both related and unrelated to their glucose lowering effects). The risk of hypoglycemia is low with this medication class. Common side effects include genital infections, increased frequency of urination and urinary tract infections. Less common side effects include euglycemic DKA, amputations (particularly with canagliflozin), reduced bone mineral density and increased risk of fractures, also with canagliflozin.

1.2.1.6. Thiazolidinedione (TZD)

These class of medications are selective agonist for peroxisome proliferator-activated receptors (PPAR-gamma), with resultant improvement in target cell response to insulin without affecting insulin release. In general terms, they increase glucose uptake in muscle and fat cells, essentially improving insulin sensitivity and lowering overall insulin resistance. Side effects include fluid retention and weight gain hence they are contraindicated in class III or IV heart failure (HF) or symptomatic HF of any class. Other less frequent but described side effects include bladder cancer and increased fracture risk in females. These medications can be used as monotherapy or in conjunction with other antidiabetic medications. Pioglitazone and Rosiglitazone are the widely available products in this class.

1.2.1.7. Glinides

These class of medications are similar to sulphonylureas but are short acting. They can be beneficial in older patients who may benefit from a sulphonylurea but have inconsistent eating habits as they are dosed within 30 minutes before meals. Examples are repaglinide and nateglinide.

1.2.1.8. Alpha Glucosidase Inhibitors

This class of medications act through inhibition of pancreatic amylase and intestinal brush border alpha glucosidases leading to delayed absorption of glucose and complex carbohydrates in the gut with subsequent delay in glucose dependent insulin production. 98% or more of the drug is not absorbed and acts locally. They are not recommended for use in estimated glomerular filtration rate (eGFR) less than 25mls/min or serum creatinine >2 mg/dl and used with caution in older persons. Available preparations are acarbose and miglitol. Given their mode of action, frequent side effects include flatulence, diarrhea, abdominal pain and less commonly elevated liver transaminases.

1.2.1.9. Bromocriptine

This is a dopamine agonist with modest glucose lowering effect, rarely prescribed for treatment of DM when compared to bromocriptine's frequent use for treatment of hyperprolactinemia.

Colesevelam is bile acid sequestrant, which also has a modest glucose lowering effect, rarely prescribed for the treatment of DM when compared with its routine indication for treatment of elevated LDL cholesterol. Side effects include nausea, constipation, dyspepsia and increased triglycerides.

1.2.1.10. Pramlintide

Pramlintide is a synthetic analogue of human amylin which slows gastric emptying, increases satiety and helps to improve post prandial hyperglycemia. It can only be used however in patients who are already taking bolus insulin hence making treatment regimen more complex with multiple daily injections. It is rarely used in T2DM and more often used in T1DM. Most notable side effect is nausea, vomiting, abdominal bloating and risk of pancreatitis.

1.2.1.11. Insulin

This is main medication option available for treatment of T1DM. It is used in T2DM in moderate to severe disease, often as part of dual or triple therapy options, particularly in managing uncontrolled T2DM. There are many available types of insulin products, most vary by their pharmacokinetics, specifically onset, peak and duration of action. They are often prescribed as only basal insulin or combination of basal and bolus insulin in multiple combinations. There are various types and strengths of insulin. Basal insulins are long acting, most common types are detemir, glargine (U100 and U300) and degludec (U100 and U200). Bolus insulin types are rapid acting such as glulisine, aspart, lispro or short acting (regular/soluble insulin). The only intermediate acting insulin available currently is NPH insulin. Other types include various pre- mix preparations (aspart protamine, lispro protamine, NPH/Regular), U500 concentrated regular insulin and inhaled insulin (a form of bolus insulin). U200, U300 and U500 insulins preparations are higher concentrations of insulin and are often considered for patients requiring much higher doses of U100 insulins. Insulin preparations are available in vials or insulin pen format for subcutaneous injections except for inhaled insulin. Insulin is often administered as single or multiple dose injections or continuous subcutaneous insulin infusion (CSII), otherwise known as insulin pump delivery system. Recommended starting dose is usually 0.4-0.5 units/kg/d for basal or basal/bolus insulin dosing for T2DM and 0.2-0.4 units/kg/day in divided (basal/bolus) dosing for T1DM. Hypoglycemia is a common risk that is encountered with most forms of treatment regimen for DM, especially in older individuals with complex insulin regimens hence efforts must be made to educate the patient on preventing, recognizing symptoms and signs, as well as appropriate treatment with glucose

1.3. Chronic Diabetic Complications and Management

Optimum glycemic control has been shown to slow down and lower risk of microvascular complications. Microvascular complications include retinopathy, nephropathy and neuropathy. Globally, diabetic retinopathy accounts for about 2·6% of all blindness and age-standardized prevalence of retinopathy as a cause of blindness was found to be highest in sub-Saharan Africa, at 0·14% [13]. In 2013 systematic review by Burges et al, the prevalence of diabetic retinopathy in sub-Saharan Africa was 30·2–31·6% and 0·9–1·3% for proliferative diabetic retinopathy, as well as 1·2–4·5% for any maculopathy. These are similar to the prevalence of these conditions worldwide with no reported differences between developed and underdeveloped countries [12, 13]. T1DM patients should be screened for retinopathy at 5 years after diagnosis, while screening for T2DM should be at the time of diagnosis. Efforts should be made to optimize glycemic control to lower risk and slow down progression of diabetic retinopathy and, when indicated, patients should be referred to ophthalmology for eye care. Treatment options for proliferative diabetic retinopathy include laser photocoagulation treatments, anti-vascular endothelial growth factor (anti-VGEF) [14].

About 35-50% of patients with T2DM will eventually progress to develop various stages of kidney damage ranging from microalbuminuria to CKD [15]. African Americans have twice the risk of end-stage renal disease compared with people of European descent, even after correction for socioeconomic and clinical risk factors. This increased risk appears to be due in part to inheritance of an apolipoprotein L1 (*APOL1*) gene variant, of which the high prevalence in West Africa might have been driven by selection for the protection it confers against some variants of trypanosomiasis [16]. Serum creatinine/eGFR and urine microalbumin creatinine ratio should be monitored annually in all diabetics, starting at 5 years after diagnosis for T1DM and at time of diagnosis for T2DM or T1DM, if diagnosed after age 30. Angiotensin-converting enzyme (ACE) inhibitors or angiotensin receptor blockers (ARB) should be used for albuminuria and efforts should be made to optimize not only glucose control but also control of blood pressure. Patients should be referred to nephrology for rapidly progressing albuminuria, deterioration in renal function or CKD stage 3.

Diabetic peripheral neuropathy is probably the most common complication of diabetes globally, affecting more than 50% of patients with diabetes [17]. In the United States, the prevalence of diabetic foot ulcers is estimated to be about 8% of patients with diabetes [17], and is higher in sub-Saharan Africa, 15% in Tanzania [18], 13% in Cameroon [19], 9.5% in Nigeria [20]. Assessment for diabetic neuropathy should commence at 5 years after diagnosis in T1DM and at time of diagnosis in T2DM. This includes foot exams, monofilament and vibration testing. Optimal glycemic control has been shown to decrease the progression of neuropathy. Severe pain symptoms may need pharmacotherapy with various classes of medications such as amitriptyline, duloxetine, gabapentin or pregabalin.

Macrovascular complications of diabetes mellitus include coronary artery disease, cerebrovascular disease and peripheral vascular disease. Overall, diabetes mellitus is a multisystemic disease with potential for significant morbidity and high disease burden, if not well controlled. Other common coexisting comorbidities such as hypertension, hyperlipidemia, obesity and obstructive sleep apnea will also need to be concurrently addressed to effectively lower overall risk of mortality. In the presence of multiple challenges as health illiteracy, access to care, poor socioeconomic status, cultural practices, lack of glucose monitoring devices and inadequate availability of multidisciplinary specialist care, it is imperative that all efforts are made on the part of the government/health care institutions, health care providers, patient, caregivers and family to achieve the diabetic individualized treatment goals.

2. Hyperthyroidism

Primary hyperthyroidism will mostly be discussed in this section. Secondary hyperthyroidism is caused by excess production of TSH from the pituitary gland resulting in increased secretion of thyroid hormone from the thyroid gland. This is exceedingly rare. Thyrotoxicosis is a disease state characterized by excess thyroid hormone presence in tissues and hyperthyroidism is a term reserved for thyrotoxicosis caused by excess thyroid hormone production. In the United States, the prevalence of hyperthyroidism is approximately 1.2% (0.5% overt and 0.7% subclinical) [21]. Blacks are often underrepresented in population based studies hence the true prevalence of hyperthyroidism is not well established in this group. Globally, prevalence is higher in regions with iodine deficiency. More broadly, subclinical hyperthyroidism can affect up to 10% of the population depending on the TSH cut-off value for defining the condition and the iodine intake of the population [22]. Common causes of hyperthyroidism include graves disease (GD), toxic multinodular goiter (TMG), and toxic adenoma (TA) [20]. Other less common causes include the thyrotoxic phase of various types of thyroiditis (subacute, silent, and destructive), medication side effects and factitious thyrotoxicosis such as surreptitious use of thyroid hormone. GD is the most common etiology of thyrotoxicosis, more common in younger individuals and women. TMG and TA are more often seen in older populations but can occur at any age. GD is caused by thyroid receptor antibodies stimulating the thyrotropin receptors resulting in increased production of thyroid hormone, usually accompanied by a diffuse goiter. This is an autoimmune disease which can go into remission with or without treatment in about a quarter of cases with lifelong risk of relapse in those who do. Prevalence of TMG and TA increases with age hence is more commonly seen in older adults, especially in areas of iodine deficiency. Autonomous thyroid hormone production can occur due to activating mutations of genes that regulate follicular cell activity and thyroid hormone synthesis.

In the thyrotoxic phase of thyroiditis, there is a diffuse inflammation of the follicular cells causing release of stored peripheral thyroid hormone from the thyroid gland into the circulation. This phase typically lasts about 4-12 weeks and resolution is often followed by euthyroidism or hypothyroidism. Several medications can also cause low TSH including dopamine agonists, glucocorticoids, and biotin. Other medications can cause thyrotoxicosis such as lithium carbonate, interferon alpha and iodine-containing medications such as amiodarone.

Clinical symptoms of hyperthyroidism include palpitations, tremors, increased sweats, hyper-defecation, increased appetite and weight loss. Extrathyroidal involvement includes eye and skin organs with possible presentations such as proptosis and exophthalmos. Older patients may present with the classic apathetic thyrotoxicosis. Physical examination findings range widely from normal findings to tachycardia, palpable goiter or thyroid nodules. A tender thyroid gland may be noted in subacute thyroiditis. Older adults may be asymptomatic or present for the first time with cardiac arrhythmias or bone loss.

In overt hyperthyroidism, TSH is low to suppressed in presence of elevated peripheral thyroid hormones (T4 and/or T3) while in subclinical hyperthyroidism, T4 and T3 are normal. Anti-TSH receptor antibodies (TRAB), thyroid-stimulating immunoglobulins (TSI) are antibodies often present in GD. Thyroid Ultrasound study may reveal a diffuse enlarged thyroid gland with increased vascularity in GD and nodule(s) in TA or TMG. Iodine 123 thyroid uptake and scan is useful in differentiating causes of hyperthyroidism with very low uptake in subacute/silent thyroiditis or factitious thyrotoxicosis, diffuse increased uptake in GD and patchy heterogeneous increased uptake or focal increased uptake (hot nodule) in TMG/TA.

It is important to treat hyperthyroidism (both overt and subclinical) in older individuals, as mild untreated subclinical hyperthyroid states can lead to complications such as tachycardia, cardiac arrhythmias, heart failure, osteopenia or osteoporosis [22] and excess mortality [23]. Most patients will need to be commenced on antithyroid medications such as methimazole, carbimazole or propylthiouracil. Beta blockers can be used to treat symptomatic tachycardia and tremors. Radioactive iodine 131 treatment and surgery/thyroidectomy may all be considered as permanent treatment options as well. Patients with thyroiditis may be treated with observation for asymptomatic patients. Non-steroidal anti-inflammatory agents (NSAIDs) or steroids may be useful for painful thyroiditis.

3. Hypothyroidism

Hypothyroidism is a common endocrine disorder resulting from deficiency of thyroid hormone. It usually is a primary process in which the thyroid gland is unable to produce enough thyroid hormone. Secondary and tertiary hypothyroidism (central) caused by TSH and TRH deficiency respectively are very uncommon. In the United States and other areas of adequate iodine intake, autoimmune thyroid disease (Hashimoto disease) is the most common cause of hypothyroidism. Worldwide, iodine deficiency is the most common cause of hypothyroidism. Hypothyroidism is more common in females compared to males. Drugs that can also cause hypothyroidism in older adults include amiodarone, interferon-α, lithium and antiepileptic drugs. Iatrogenic causes include thyroidectomy, radioactive iodine treatment and external beam radiation therapy. Causes of central hypothyroidism include: pituitary adenomas, sarcoidosis, tuberculous meningitis, and brain radiation.

3.1. Prevalence

Hypothyroidism increases in prevalence and incidence with increasing age. The prevalence of overt hypothyroidism in the general population ranges between 0.2% and 5.3% in Europe and 0.3%-3.7% in the United States [24]. The overall disease burden of hypothyroidism in sub-Saharan Africa, based largely on hospital clinical data, is predicted to be minimal (or even rare) and substantially lower than the prevalence found in African Americans [25]. There is growing evidence that normal TSH distribution curves appear to be shifted towards higher value ranges in older individuals. Very mild TSH elevations in older individuals may not reflect subclinical thyroid dysfunction but rather be a normal consequence of ageing [26]. Older adults, 80 years and above, have higher TSH levels in all races, while Caucasians tend to have higher TSH readings than African American across all ages.

3.2. Clinical Presentation and Management

Presentation of overt hypothyroidism in the older person is varied, non-specific, and often insidious. Older people with hypothyroidism report fewer symptoms compared to younger counterparts [27]. Some of these classic symptoms are more likely to be misattributed to other co-morbid conditions or a manifestation of the aging process. Symptoms include fatigue, cold intolerance, weight gain, constipation, arthralgias. Physical findings evident in hypothyroid older individuals may include bradycardia, diastolic hypertension, pallor, dry skin, coarse hair, hoarseness, dysarthria, delayed relaxation of deep tendon reflexes, and mental status changes [28]. Myxedema coma is a severe form of hypothyroidism that results in an altered mental status, hypothermia, bradycardia, hypercarbia, and hyponatremia. Cardiomegaly, pericardial effusion, cardiogenic shock, and ascites may also be present. Most patients presenting with myxedema coma are older adults. Severe medical complications of hypothyroidism are more common in affected older persons.

Diagnosis is made with an elevated TSH for primary hypothyroidism. Subclinical hypothyroidism is common in this population and is characterized by an elevated TSH in the presence of normal free thyroid hormones. In cases of suspected central hypothyroidism that may result from disruption of the anatomy or function of the hypothalamic-pituitary axis, the TSH level may not be relied upon as an accurate index of thyroid function. In this setting the free T4 level may serve as more reliable measure of thyroid hormone production.

For management of hypothyroidism, international guidelines suggest a TSH cutoff of 10 mIU/L and repeating within 3 to 6 months before treatment, is recommended [29]. Initial treatment of hypothyroidism in older patients should typically start with levothyroxine (thyroxine) administered in lower doses than those usually prescribed for healthy younger patients. Once cardiovascular tolerance of a starting dose has been assessed, most experts recommend gradually increasing daily doses by 12.5-25 mcg every four to six weeks until adequate replacement is confirmed by repeat TSH measurement. An optimal TSH target value should be ~2.5 to 3.5 mIU/L [28]. A normal Free T4 level is the goal for treating central hypothyroidism. The dose of levothyroxine that normalizes serum TSH level is lower in older patients due to changes in thyroxine turnover with age related reduction in lean body mass. Other factors such as decreased absorption, concomitant medication use, and other comorbidities could also affect thyroid hormone metabolism [30]. Ensuring compliance with therapy is essential to avoid unnecessary levothyroxine dose increase. Overtreatment with excessive doses of thyroxine may be associated with significant morbidity in older adults. Exposure to excessive amounts of thyroid hormone may be associated with increased risks of atrial fibrillation, other tachyarrhythmias, and progressive decline in bone mineral density [31].

4. Thyroid Nodules and Thyroid Cancer

Thyroid nodules are more frequent in older adult patients, with a linear increase with age in both the presence of nodules and the absolute number of nodules per patient [32]. This is partly related to the increased use of high-frequency ultrasound, CT, and MR imaging in routine clinical care, leading to the detection of asymptomatic, or incidental, thyroid nodules [32]. Measurement of thyroid stimulating hormone (TSH) and imaging with thyroid ultrasound are invaluable in the evaluation of thyroid nodules. If the TSH is low, further evaluation for a functioning nodule is warranted. Risk factors for thyroid cancer include prior head and neck irradiation, family history, low iodine diet (for Follicular cancers), thyroid cancer syndromes. Fine needle aspiration (FNA) biopsy is the recommended modality for sampling thyroid nodules. Cytology specimens collected by FNA are classified traditionally by the Bethesda System for Reporting Thyroid Cytopathology. This is a challenge in countries where there are limited resources available. Thyroid cancer is present in 4-6.5% of thyroid nodules. The four main types of thyroid cancers are papillary, follicular, medullary and anaplastic, with the first two referred to as differentiated thyroid cancer (DTC). Thyroid cancer incidence varies by race/ethnicity. According to the United States National Cancer Institute's Surveillance, Epidemiology, and End Results Program (SEER-18) database, from 2000-2014, whites had the highest estimated thyroid cancer incidence rate followed by Hispanics, Asians, Native Americans, and African Americans [33]. The documented prevalence rates of thyroid cancer in the African continent in one study are as follows: papillary: 6.7–72.1%, follicular: 4.9–68%, anaplastic: 5–21.4%, and medullary: 2.6%–13.8%. For DTC, there is a changing trend toward the more frequent occurrence of papillary thyroid cancer (PTC) compared to follicular thyroid cancer (FTC) and this may be attributable to widespread iodization programs [34]. FTC is still common in developing countries, whereas PTC is the predominant subtype in developed countries. Thyroid cancer continues to present with a high female predominance. Some studies show a pattern of more widespread disease at presentation in older adult patients and a relative increase in the frequency of more aggressive histologic subtypes.

The cornerstones of therapy for DTC are surgical resection, radioactive iodine (RAI) ablation, and thyroid hormone suppression of TSH. Serum thyroglobulin trends and follow-up neck ultrasound imaging are used for monitoring patients over time. However, older adult patients are more likely to receive thyroidectomy at community and low-volume sites, where the rate of surgical complications may be higher [35]. For diagnosed thyroid cancer, surgical resection is generally recommended as a primary form of treatment in most cases. However, in a low-resource setting, the degree of thyroid resection should be carefully considered in light of how the extent of thyroid surgery may influence perioperative complications and long-term quality of life. Generally, patients in the American Thyroid Association (ATA) high and intermediate risk category should be considered for RAI therapy to ablate residual disease and remnant thyroid tissue [35]. Individualized targets for TSH suppression in thyroid cancer is recommended, generally targeting a low to low-normal range TSH. Greater TSH suppression in more aggressive disease is balanced with greater cardiac and bone complications in older adult patients [36]. Older adults on chronic suppressive levothyroxine therapy, are also at risk for bone loss and fractures. In addition, older patients are more likely to have co-morbid cardiac disease, including arrhythmias, coronary artery disease, and heart failure, which can place them at increased risk for complications from thyroid hormone excess. Currently two tyrosine kinase inhibitors are approved for therapy of metastatic, radio-resistant differentiated thyroid cancer: sorafenib and lenvatinib.

5. OSTEOPOROSIS

Osteoporosis is characterized by low bone mass, skeletal fragility and microarchitectural disruption. It usually has no clinical manifestations until there is a fracture. It is a major public health problem; and is often unrecognized and untreated. Women have about an 80% higher rate of osteoporotic fractures than men after adjusting for age. Hip fractures carry a significant risk of increased morbidity and mortality. As sub-Saharan Africa undergoes an epidemiological transition as a result of rapid urbanization, the burden of non-communicable diseases, including osteoporosis, is rising [37]. Decreased bone mineral density (BMD) is associated with increased risk of fracture in both older black and white women. It has been reported that African American women have higher BMD and lower fracture risk than Caucasian women [38]. Although postmenopausal African American women are at lower risk for osteoporosis-related fractures compared with white women, fractures in African American women are associated with significantly higher morbidity and mortality. Therefore, early diagnosis and treatment of osteoporosis in this population is just as important as it is for other ethnic groups. Epidemiological studies reporting the incidence of hip fracture or vertebral fractures are limited from Africa, especially sub-Saharan Africa. Fewer African American women receive dual energy X-ray absorptiometry (DXA) screenings and are treated for osteoporosis [39]. A clinical diagnosis of osteoporosis can be made in the presence of a fragility fracture or a T score of -2.5 standard deviations (SDs) or lower in the lumbar spine (anteroposterior), femoral neck, total hip, or 1/3 radius based upon bone mineral density measured by DXA. A diagnosis of Osteopenia is made when the T score is between -1.0 to -2.5. Patients with osteopenia and a high fracture risk assessment tool (FRAX) score also have a high risk for fracture. The FRAX score is considered high if the risk of a major osteoporotic fracture is 20% and that of a hip fracture is 3%. Clinical risk factors in FRAX® include age, sex, body mass index (BMI), smoking, alcohol use, prior fracture, parental history of hip fracture, use of glucocorticoids, rheumatoid arthritis, secondary osteoporosis, and femoral neck BMD, when available. Trabecular bone score, an indirect measure of bone structure, may differ between ethnicities. It has been noted that African Americans had lower trabecular bone score than do Caucasians referred for densitometry, even when controlling for age and abdominal soft tissue thickness.

Secondary causes of osteoporosis include diabetes mellitus, hyperparathyroidism, hyperthyroidism, chronic liver disease, malabsorption syndromes, vitamin D deficiency, rheumatoid arthritis, renal failure, HIV and chronic liver disease. High risk drugs for osteoporosis include corticosteroids, aromatase inhibitors, proton pump inhibitors, pioglitazone, selective serotonin reuptake inhibitors (SSRI) and canagliflozin (SGLT-2 Inhibitor). A thorough evaluation for secondary causes is required. Initial testing includes complete blood count, basic metabolic panel, liver function tests, 25-OH vitamin D, phosphate, 24-hour urine collection for calcium [40]. Further testing could be necessary depending on the clinical situation and may include intact PTH, TSH, celiac disease panel and serum protein electrophoresis.

Non- Pharmacologic therapy for osteoporosis includes counseling patients to maintain adequate dietary intake of calcium, up to a total dietary intake and supplements (if needed) of 1,200 mg/day. Supplementation with Vitamin D3, with a daily dose of 1,000 to 2,000 international units (IU) is typically required to maintain an optimal serum 25-OH vitamin D level [40]. Higher doses of vitamin D supplementation maybe needed in some clinical instances. Prevalence of vitamin D deficiency in Africa is high [41]. There is a higher prevalence of lactase deficiency in African Americans and some parts of Africa which affects the amount of calcium absorbed in the diets. Weight bearing and balance exercises, fall precautions, smoking cessation, limitation of alcohol consumption are very important factors to consider in these patients. Candidates for pharmacologic therapy are patients with osteoporosis, fragility fractures (irrespective of BMD) osteopenia with high FRAX score. Pharmacologic therapy include: antiresorptive agents such as alendronate, denosumab, risedronate, zoledronate and anabolic agents such as abaloparatide, teriparatide, romosozumab. Abaloparatide, denosumab, romosozumab, teriparatide, and zoledronate should be considered for patients unable to use oral therapy and as initial therapy for patients at very high fracture risk [40]. Duration of treatment and consideration for drug holiday depends on the agent used and also the risk of fracture. Patients on treatment need to be monitored with serial BMD testing. This could be done every 1-2 years but less frequently when bone density is stable. Serial monitoring is based on absolute BMD and not T-scores. The goal of monitoring osteoporosis therapy is to identify those who have significant bone loss. In patients on treatment, stable or increasing BMD at the spine and hip indicates a satisfactory response.

6. Hyperparathyroidism

Parathyroid organ system consist of bilateral sets of superior and inferior small glands located posterior to the thyroid gland. Occasionally, there could be an ectopic or misplaced parathyroid gland. Parathyroid hormone (PTH) is the hormone secreted from the parathyroid glands to regulate calcium metabolism through its actions in the kidney and bones. Below are common parathyroid disorders with increasing prevalence with age.

6.1. Primary Hyperparathyroidism (PHP)

PHP is an endocrine disorder characterized by hypercalcemia in the setting of inappropriately elevated serum PTH. Causes include parathyroid adenoma (often involves 1 gland), parathyroid hyperplasia (often involves multiple glands), and very rarely parathyroid carcinoma. PHP is caused by a solitary parathyroid adenoma in 80% of cases, whereas four-gland hyperplasia accounts for 10–15%, multiple adenomas for 5% and parathyroid cancer for <1% of cases [42]. Normocalcemic PHP can sometimes occur, few of these patients can progress over several years to developing hypercalcemic PHP but majority remain normocalcemic. Incidence of PHP complications such as bone loss, fractures and renal stones are still significant, as with the hypercalcemic variant [43]. The incidence of

PHP increases with age and is higher in women and African Americans than other racial groups [44]. In general, lower vitamin D, higher PTH levels and lower risk of osteoporotic fractures have been described as inherently prevalent in blacks when compared with other races. These distinctive features of calcium homeostasis in this racial group have raised questions regarding whether the established normal range for vitamin D is appropriate for blacks [45-47]. Most cases of PHP are discovered incidentally with elevated serum calcium during routine lab draws or elevated intact PTH levels during routine work up for osteoporosis. Less often, this is discovered during work up for other conditions such as renal stones, multiple endocrine neoplasia type 1(MEN1) and other related genetic/familial disorders. Symptomatic presentation is still relatively more common in African countries due to lack of routine laboratory screening which would have picked up cases earlier than onset of symptoms. Common symptoms include bone pain, fatigue and abdominal pain. Common laboratory findings in PHP include elevated serum calcium (total or ionized or both), inappropriately elevated PTH, low or low normal serum phosphorus, calculated fractional excretion of calcium more than 1%. Other findings include low or low normal 25-OH vitamin D, high or high normal 1,25-OH vitamin D (on account of increased 1-alpha-hydroxylase enzyme activity) and normal or elevated serum alkaline phosphatase (ALP) from compensatory increased bone formation to PTH induced increased bone resorption. It is important that PTH levels are measured using a PTH intact (second generation) assay or a third generation assay rather than a first generation PTH assay which traditionally would cross-react with PTH- related peptide (PTH-RP) making it unable to distinguish elevated PTH from PHP vs elevated PTH RP in hypercalcemia of malignancy. Parathyroid imaging is not necessary for making a diagnosis but usually helpful to the surgeon in localizing the affected gland if the patient will undergo surgical parathyroidectomy. A bone density study may reveal bone loss especially in cortical sites, hence it is wise to include distal forearm to traditional lumbar spine and hip sites for BMD measurements.

Treatment for PHP can be medical or surgical. Surgery should be considered in all symptomatic and asymptomatic patients that meet guideline for surgical management. The indications for surgical management [48] include: serum calcium more than 1.0 mg/dl higher than upper limit of normal levels, vertebral fractures or T score in BMD below -2.5, hypercalciuria (24-hour urine calcium >400) or renal stones, renal failure with eGFR <60 (other cofounding factors such as age and comorbidities like hypertension or diabetes may contribute to this), age less than 50 years, and expected difficulty in long term monitoring. Other considerations for surgical management with weak recommendations and low quality evidence include: neuropsychiatric/neurocognitive symptoms, cardiovascular disease, muscle weakness, and gastroesophageal reflux symptoms. Risk of post-operative complications is lower in well experienced parathyroid surgeons. Medical management can be considered in patients who do not meet surgical criteria, have high surgical risk or do not want surgery. Medical treatment options are limited and include: cinacalcet, which could help normalize serum calcium and may/may not improve PTH level and bisphosphonate therapy to treat bone loss or osteoporosis. Patients who fall into the category of long term follow up usually exhibit fairly stable parameters but studies have shown that BMD starts to decline at cortical sites before 10 years and 37% of patients develop one or more indications for parathyroidectomy over 15 years of follow-up [49]. These patients should have annual laboratory monitoring with serum chemistries, calcium, renal function, alkaline phosphatase, phosphorus, 25 OH vitamin D and 24-hour urine calcium. Bone density scans should be performed every 2 years.

6.2. Secondary Hyperparathyroidism (SHP)

SHP is often found in chronic kidney disease characterized by elevated PTH level in the setting of normal or low calcium, elevated phosphorus and often low vitamin D levels. This is usually addressed by renal specialist as part of broad management of chronic kidney diseases and is discussed in the chapter on kidney diseases in older adults. SHP could also however be temporarily seen in isolated vitamin D deficiency without CKD and this tends to reverse once vitamin D stores are repleted.

6.3. Tertiary Hyperparathyroidism (THP)

THP is also a complication of end stage renal disease often seen in patients already undergoing renal replacement therapy and typically managed by renal specialist as part of broad management of chronic kidney diseases. Parathyroid carcinomas are very rare and account for less than one percent of PHP, so will not be discussed in detail in this chapter.

7. Adrenal Nodules

Adrenal nodules are often found as incidentalomas on routine abdominal imaging studies performed for non-adrenal related indications. Incidence of imaging studies and thus incidentalomas increase with age, especially in developed countries hence these can be quite commonly seen and are often benign. Radiological characteristics of the nodules can distinguish between benign and malignant lesions. All adrenal nodules should undergo hormonal evaluation to screen for Cushing's syndrome, pheochromocytoma and primary hyperaldosteronism (in patients with hypertension).

8. Pituitary Tumors

These can also be found incidentally on brain imaging studies performed for other indications. Patients may present with clinical picture of any of the pituitary hormonal deficiency or excesses or less often features consistent with compression of tumor to surrounding structures. Patients should undergo pituitary hormonal evaluation and treatment as necessary, for any diagnosed hormonal deficiency or excesses. Appropriate long term tumor follow up is also indicated in patients who do not require surgical management.

REFERENCES

[1] Carlsson S. Etiology and Pathogenesis of Latent Autoimmune Diabetes in Adults (LADA) Compared to Type 2 Diabetes. *Front Physiol.* 2019; 10:320. Published 2019 Mar 26. doi: 10.3389/fphys. 2019.00320.

[2] Vellanki P, Umpierrez GE. Diabetic ketoacidosis: A common debut of Diabetes among African Americans with Type 2 Diabetes. *Endocr Pract.* 2017; 23(8):971-978.

[3] Saeedi P, Petersohn I, Salpea P, Malanda B, Karuranga S, Unwin N, Colagiuri S, Guariguata L, Motala AA, Ogurtsova K, Shaw JE, Bright D, Williams R; IDF Diabetes Atlas Committee. Global and regional diabetes prevalence estimates for 2019 and projections for 2030 and 2045: Results from the International Diabetes Federation Diabetes Atlas, 9th edition. *Diabetes Res Clin Pract.* 2019 Nov; 157:107843.

[4] United Nations Department of Economic and Social Affairs. *World Population Ageing 2019.* Available at: https://www.un.org/en/development/desa/population/publications/pdf/ageing/WorldPopulationAgeing2019-Highlights.pdf. Accessed December 11,2020.

[5] Xu G, Liu B, Sun Y, Du Y, Snetselaar LG, Hu FB, Bao W. Prevalence of diagnosed type 1 and type 2 diabetes among US adults in 2016 and 2017: population based study. *BMJ.* 2018 Sep 4; 362:k1497.

[6] Fang M. Trends in the Prevalence of Diabetes Among U.S. Adults: 1999-2016. *Am J Prev Med.* 2018 Oct; 55(4):497-505.

[7] Werfalli M, Kassanjee R, Kalula S, Kowal P, Phaswana-Mafuya N, Levitt NS. Diabetes in South African older adults: prevalence and impact on quality of life and functional disability - as assessed using SAGE Wave 1 data. *Glob Health Action.* 2018; 11(1):1449924.

[8] Mohamed SF, Mwangi M, Mutua MK, Kibachio J, Hussein A, Ndegwa Z, Owondo S, Asiki G, Kyobutungi C. Prevalence and factors associated with pre-diabetes and diabetes mellitus in Kenya: results from a national survey. *BMC Public Health.* 2018 Nov 7; 18(Suppl 3):1215.

[9] Uloko AE, Musa BM, Ramalan MA, Gezawa ID, Puepet FH, Uloko AT, Borodo MM, Sada KB. Prevalence and Risk Factors for Diabetes Mellitus in Nigeria: A Systematic Review and Meta-Analysis. *Diabetes Ther.* 2018 Jun; 9(3):1307-1316.

[10] LeRoith D, Biessels GJ, Braithwaite SS, Casanueva FF, Draznin B, Halter JB et al. Treatment of Diabetes in Older Adults: An Endocrine Society* Clinical Practice Guideline. *J Clin Endocrinol Metab.* 2019; 104(5):1520-1574.

[11] Carlsson S. Etiology and Pathogenesis of Latent Autoimmune Diabetes in Adults (LADA) Compared to Type 2 Diabetes. *Front Physiol.* 2019 Mar 26; 10:320.

[12] Burgess PI, MacCormick IJ, Harding SP, Bastawrous A, Beare NA, Garner P. Epidemiology of diabetic retinopathy and maculopathy in Africa: a systematic review. *Diabet Med.* 2013 Apr; 30(4):399-412.

[13] Atun R, Davies JI, Gale EAM, Bärnighausen T, Beran D et al. Diabetes in sub-Saharan Africa: from clinical care to health policy. *Lancet Diabetes Endocrinol.* 2017 Aug; 5(8):622-667.

[14] Wang W, Lo ACY. Diabetic Retinopathy: Pathophysiology and Treatments. *Int J Mol Sci.* 2018 Jun 20; 19(6):1816.

[15] Fu H, Liu S, Bastacky SI, Wang X, Tian XJ, Zhou D. Diabetic kidney diseases revisited: A new perspective for a new era. *Mol Metab.* 2019 Dec; 30:250-263.

[16] Genovese G, Friedman DJ, Ross MD, Lecordier L, Uzureau P, Freedman BI, Bowden DW, Langefeld CD, Oleksyk TK, Uscinski Knob AL, Bernhardy AJ, Hicks PJ, Nelson GW, Vanhollebeke B, Winkler CA, Kopp JB, Pays E, Pollak MR. Association of trypanolytic ApoL1 variants with kidney disease in African Americans. *Science.* 2010 Aug 13; 329(5993):841-5.

[17] Abbas ZG. The global burden of diabetic foot. In: Pendsey S (ed) *Contemporary management of diabetic foot, Jaypee Brothers Medical Publishers*, New Delhi 2014: 24-3.0.

[18] Abbas ZG, Lutale JK, Bakker K, Baker N, Archibald LK. The 'Step by Step' Diabetic Foot Project in Tanzania: a model for improving patient outcomes in less-developed countries. *Int Wound J.* 2011; 8(2):169-175.

[19] Ndip EA, Tchakonte B, Mbanya JC. A study of the prevalence and risk factors of foot problems in a population of diabetic patients in cameroon. *Int J Low Extrem Wounds.* 2006 Jun; 5(2):83-8.

[20] Ogbera AO, Fasanmade O, Ohwovoriole AE, Adediran O. An assessment of the disease burden of foot ulcers in patients with diabetes mellitus attending a teaching hospital in Lagos, Nigeria. *Int J Low Extrem Wounds.* 2006 Dec; 5(4):244-9.

[21] Ross DS, Burch HB, Cooper DS, Greenlee MC, Laurberg P, Maia AL, Rivkees SA, Samuels M, Sosa JA, Stan MN, Walter MA. 2016 American Thyroid Association Guidelines for Diagnosis and Management of Hyperthyroidism and Other Causes of Thyrotoxicosis. *Thyroid.* 2016 Oct; 26(10):1343-1421.

[22] Carlé A, Andersen SL, Boelaert K, Laurberg P. Management Of Endocrine Disease: Subclinical thyrotoxicosis: prevalence, causes and choice of therapy. *Eur J Endocrinol.* 2017 Jun; 176(6):R325-R337.

[23] Grossman A, Weiss A, Koren-Morag N, Shimon I, Beloosesky Y, Meyerovitch J. Subclinical Thyroid Disease and Mortality in the Elderly: A Retrospective Cohort Study. *Am J Med.* 2016 Apr; 129(4):423-30.

[24] Chaker L, Bianco AC, Jonklaas J, Peeters RP. Hypothyroidism. *Lancet.* 2017 Sep 23; 390(10101):1550-1562.

[25] Taylor PN, Albrecht D, Scholz A, Gutierrez-Buey G, Lazarus JH, Dayan CM, Okosieme OE. Global epidemiology of hyperthyroidism and hypothyroidism. *Nat Rev Endocrinol.* 2018 May; 14(5):301-316.

[26] Jonklaas J, Razvi S. Reference intervals in the diagnosis of thyroid dysfunction: treating patients not numbers. *Lancet Diabetes Endocrinol.* 2019 Jun; 7(6):473-483.

[27] Carlé A, Pedersen IB, Knudsen N, Perrild H, Ovesen L, Andersen S, Laurberg P. Hypothyroid Symptoms Fail to Predict Thyroid Insufficiency in Old People: A Population-Based Case-Control Study. *Am J Med*. 2016 Oct; 129(10):1082-92.

[28] Mokshagundam S, Barzel US. Thyroid disease in the elderly. *J Am Geriatr Soc*. 1993 Dec; 41(12):1361-9.

[29] Jonklaas J, Bianco AC, Bauer AJ, Burman KD, Cappola AR, Celi FS, Cooper DS, Kim BW, Peeters RP, Rosenthal MS, Sawka AM; American Thyroid Association Task Force on Thyroid Hormone Replacement. Guidelines for the treatment of hypothyroidism: prepared by the American Thyroid Association task force on thyroid hormone replacement. *Thyroid*. 2014 Dec; 24(12):1670-751.

[30] Leng O, Razvi S. Hypothyroidism in the older population. *Thyroid Res*. 2019 Feb 8; 12:2.

[31] Flynn RW, Bonellie SR, Jung RT, MacDonald TM, Morris AD, Leese GP. Serum thyroid-stimulating hormone concentration and morbidity from cardiovascular disease and fractures in patients on long-term thyroxine therapy. *J Clin Endocrinol Metab*. 2010 Jan; 95(1):186-93

[32] Kwong N, Medici M, Angell TE, Liu X, Marqusee E, Cibas ES, Krane JF, Barletta JA, Kim MI, Larsen PR, Alexander EK. The Influence of Patient Age on Thyroid Nodule Formation, Multinodularity, and Thyroid Cancer Risk. *J Clin Endocrinol Metab*. 2015 Dec; 100(12):4434-40.

[33] Weeks KS, Kahl AR, Lynch CF, Charlton ME. Racial/ethnic differences in thyroid cancer incidence in the United States, 2007-2014. *Cancer*. 2018 Apr 1; 124(7):1483-1491.

[34] Ogbera AO, Kuku SF. Epidemiology of thyroid diseases in Africa. *Indian J Endocrinol Metab*. 2011 Jul; 15(Suppl 2):S82-8.

[35] Sosa JA, Mehta PJ, Wang TS, Boudourakis L, Roman SA. A population-based study of outcomes from thyroidectomy in aging Americans: at what cost? *J Am Coll Surg*. 2008 Jun; 206(6):1097-105.

[36] Haugen BR, Alexander EK, Bible KC, Doherty GM, Mandel SJ et al. 2015 American Thyroid Association Management Guidelines for Adult Patients with Thyroid Nodules and Differentiated Thyroid

Cancer: The American Thyroid Association Guidelines Task Force on Thyroid Nodules and Differentiated Thyroid Cancer. *Thyroid.* 2016 Jan; 26(1):1-133.

[37] Gregson CL, Cassim B, Micklesfield LK, Lukhele M, Ferrand RA, Ward KA; SAMSON Collaborative Working Group. Fragility fractures in sub-Saharan Africa: time to break the myth. *Lancet Glob Health.* 2019 Jan; 7(1):e26-e27.

[38] Cauley JA, Lui LY, Ensrud KE, Zmuda JM, Stone KL, Hochberg MC, Cummings SR. Bone mineral density and the risk of incident nonspinal fractures in black and white women. *JAMA.* 2005 May 4; 293 (17):2102-8.

[39] Hamrick I, Cao Q, Agbafe-Mosley D, Cummings DM. Osteoporosis healthcare disparities in postmenopausal women. *J Womens Health* (Larchmt). 2012 Dec; 21(12):1232-6.

[40] Camacho PM, Petak SM, Binkley N, Diab DL, Eldeiry LS, Farooki A, Harris ST, Hurley DL, Kelly J, Lewiecki EM, Pessah-Pollack R, Mcclung M, Wimalawansa SJ, Watts NB. American Association of Clinical Endocrinologists/American College of Endocrinology Clinical Practice Guidelines for the Diagnosis and Treatment of Postmenopausal Osteoporosis-2020 Update. *Endocr Pract.* 2020 May; 26(Suppl 1):1-46.

[41] Mogire RM, Mutua A, Kimita W, Kamau A, Bejon P, Pettifor JM, Adeyemo A, Williams TN, Atkinson SH. Prevalence of vitamin D deficiency in Africa: a systematic review and meta-analysis. *Lancet Glob Health.* 2020 Jan; 8(1):e134-e142.

[42] Walker MD, Silverberg SJ. Primary hyperparathyroidism. *Nat Rev Endocrinol.* 2018 Feb; 14(2):115-125.

[43] Tuna MM, Çalışkan M, Ünal M, Demirci T, Doğan BA, Küçükler K, Özbek M, Berker D, Delibaşı T, Güler S. Normocalcemic hyperparathyroidism is associated with complications similar to those of hypercalcemic hyperparathyroidism. *J Bone Miner Metab.* 2016 May; 34(3):331-5.

[44] Yeh MW, Ituarte PH, Zhou HC, Nishimoto S, Liu IL, Harari A, Haigh PI, Adams AL. Incidence and prevalence of primary

hyperparathyroidism in a racially mixed population. *J Clin Endocrinol Metab.* 2013 Mar; 98(3):1122-9.

[45] Wright NC, Chen L, Niu J, Neogi T, Javiad K, Nevitt MA, Lewis CE, Curtis JR. Defining physiologically "normal" vitamin D in African Americans. *Osteoporos Int.* 2012 Sep; 23(9):2283-91.

[46] Golden SH, Brown A, Cauley JA, Chin MH, Gary-Webb TL, Kim C, Sosa JA, Sumner AE, Anton B. Health disparities in endocrine disorders: biological, clinical, and nonclinical factors--an Endocrine Society scientific statement. *J Clin Endocrinol Metab.* 2012 Sep; 97(9):E1579-639.

[47] Cauley JA, Danielson ME, Boudreau R, Barbour KE, Horwitz MJ, Bauer DC, Ensrud KE, Manson JE, Wactawski-Wende J, Shikany JM, Jackson RD. Serum 25-hydroxyvitamin D and clinical fracture risk in a multiethnic cohort of women: the Women's Health Initiative (WHI). *J Bone Miner Res.* 2011 Oct; 26(10):2378-88.

[48] Wilhelm SM, Wang TS, Ruan DT, Lee JA, Asa SL, Duh QY, Doherty GM, Herrera MF, Pasieka JL, Perrier ND, Silverberg SJ, Solórzano CC, Sturgeon C, Tublin ME, Udelsman R, Carty SE. The American Association of Endocrine Surgeons Guidelines for Definitive Management of Primary Hyperparathyroidism. *JAMA Surg.* 2016 Oct 1;151(10):959-968.

[49] Rubin MR, Bilezikian JP, McMahon DJ, Jacobs T, Shane E, Siris E, Udesky J, Silverberg SJ. The natural history of primary hyperparathyroidism with or without parathyroid surgery after 15 years. *J Clin Endocrinol Metab.* 2008 Sep; 93(9):3462-70.

In: Care of the Older African Adult
Editor: Seki A. Balogun
ISBN: 978-1-53619-295-7

Chapter 11

GASTROINTESTINAL DISORDERS IN OLDER ADULTS OF AFRICAN DESCENT

Omar Massoud[1,*], Mohamed Ahmed[2] and Moustafa Massoud[3]
[1]Chief, Hepatology Section,
Department of Gastroenterology and Hepatology,
Cleveland Clinic Foundation, Cleveland, Ohio
[2]Resident, Department of Internal Medicine,
University of Missouri - Kansas city
[3]Assistant Professor, Department of Internal Medicine,
University of Alabama at Birmingham, Birmingham, Alabama

ABSTRACT

The different prevalence and behavior of diseases among distinct racial cohorts has always been in question. Genetic, economic, and cultural variabilities have been examined in hopes to determine a relationship between the occurrence and severity of a disease and certain racial group.

In this chapter we review a group of the most common gastrointestinal diseases and whether there is a difference in their incidence, nature of the disease and response to treatment related to patients from African descent.

[*] Corresponding Author's Email: massouo@ccf.org.

In addition, we review if mortality rate or morbidity associated with certain gastrointestinal diseases is affected by genetic difference among different racial groups or is the difference mostly attributed to different socioeconomic statuses.

Literature yielded has been variable and while with some diseases a link could be established or rejected, other diseases do not seem to have enough data that would conclude such a link.

Keywords: gastrointestinal disease, older adults, African American, race, esophageal disease, gastric cancer, pancreatitis, pancreatic cancer, hemochromatosis

1. Achalasia

Achalasia is described as an impairment of lower esophageal sphincter (LES) relaxation and absence of peristalsis in the smooth muscle layer of the esophagus. Primary achalasia is usually idiopathic. Secondary achalasia is most commonly due to malignancy and may be attributed to diseases that cause esophageal motor abnormalities [1]. Older adults are more likely to have secondary achalasia. Achalasia results from inflammation and degeneration of neurons in the esophageal wall. Although this is most commonly idiopathic, there are observations connecting achalasia to variants in the HLA-DQ region which suggests that affected patients may have circulating antibodies against specific neurons [2, 3]. This genetic predisposition is seen in syndromes such as Allgrove syndrome with achalasia, alacrima, and adrenal insufficiency.

The clinical manifestations of achalasia consist of dysphagia, regurgitation, chest pain, hiccups, halitosis, weight loss, and aspiration pneumonia [4]. Achalasia should be suspected in patients with dysphagia to solids and liquids, heartburn resistant to PPI, retained food seen on upper endoscopy, and increased resistance to passing the endoscope through the esophagogastric junction (EGJ). Esophageal manometry is the gold standard for diagnosis [5].

Treatment options include pneumatic balloon dilation, surgical myotomy, and botulinum toxin injection. Pneumatic balloon dilation and surgical myotomy both have a high success rate. Similarly, botulinum toxin has a high initial success rate but more frequent relapses and a shorter time to relapse when compared to balloon dilation or myotomy.

2. Gastroesophageal Reflux Disease (GERD)

Gastroesophageal reflux disease (GERD) happens as a result of the failure of the normal anti-reflux barrier to function against abnormal amounts of refluxed material. The prevalence of GERD has only recently been studied in minority populations in the United States. In a recent survey of 1172 participants at a community fair, 50% of Hispanics experienced heartburn at least monthly, compared with 37% of Caucasians, 31% of African Americans, and 20% of Asians [6].

Clinical manifestations of GERD include classic symptoms of heartburn (pyrosis) and regurgitation. Heartburn is typically described as a burning sensation in the retrosternal area, mostly experienced in the postprandial period. Heartburn is considered troublesome if mild symptoms occur two or more days a week, or moderate to severe symptoms occur more than one day a week. Regurgitation is defined as the perception of flow of refluxed gastric content into the mouth or hypopharynx. Patients typically regurgitate acidic material mixed with small amounts of undigested food. Other symptoms of GERD include dysphagia, chest pain, water brash, globus sensation, odynophagia, nausea, and extra-esophageal symptoms such as chronic cough, hoarseness, and wheezing.

2.1. Clinical Management

In patients with classic symptoms, the diagnosis of GERD can often be based on only clinical symptoms such as heartburn and/or regurgitation. However, patients may require additional evaluation if they have alarm features, risk factors for Barrett's esophagus, or abnormal gastrointestinal imaging performed for evaluation of their symptoms.

In patients without classic symptoms, other symptoms such as chest pain, globus sensation, chronic cough, hoarseness, wheezing, and nausea may be seen in the setting of GERD, but are not sufficient to make a clinical diagnosis of GERD in the absence of classic symptoms of heartburn and regurgitation. Other disorders need to be excluded before attributing the symptoms to GERD. As an example, unexplained chest pain should be evaluated with an electrocardiogram and exercise stress test prior to a gastrointestinal evaluation.

Ambulatory esophageal pH monitoring is also used to confirm the diagnosis of GERD in those with persistent symptoms (whether typical or atypical, particularly if a trial of twice-daily PPI has failed) or to monitor the adequacy of treatment in those with continued symptoms.

Upper endoscopy is indicated in patients with suspected GERD to evaluate for alarm symptoms such as odynophagia, weight loss, or unexplained anemia which may be indicative of gastrointestinal (GI) bleed. Upper endoscopy should also be performed to screen for Barrett's esophagus in patients with high risk factors. The Los Angeles classification grades esophagitis severity by the extent of mucosal abnormality, with complications recorded separately. In this grading scheme, a mucosal break refers to an area of slough adjacent to more normal mucosa in the squamous epithelium with or without overlying exudate: Grade A – One or more mucosal breaks, each $\leq$ 5 mm in length; Grade B – At least one mucosal break > 5 mm long, but not continuous between the tops of adjacent mucosal folds; Grade C – At least one mucosal break that is continuous between the tops of adjacent mucosal folds, but which is not circumferential; Grade D – Mucosal break that involves at least three-fourths of the luminal circumference.

In treating GERD, head of bed elevation and weight loss is recommended. Typically, an 8-week course of PPI daily is initiated as treatment. Patients with a refractory or incomplete response may get twice daily PPI or switching to a different PPI. If symptoms persist, then upper endoscopy is performed to exclude non-GERD etiologies.

3. Barrett's Esophagus

Barrett's esophagus (BE) is the condition in which an abnormal columnar epithelium that is predisposed to malignancy substitutes the stratified squamous epithelium that is present in the distal esophagus. In several studies, Barrett's esophagus appears to have a higher prevalence in Caucasians as compared to Hispanics and Asians, and prevalence appears to be lowest in African Americans.

An endoscopic grading system (The Prague C & M Criteria) has been recommended for reporting the extent of Barrett's esophagus. Measurements should be obtained during withdrawal of the endoscope when the shaft of the endoscope is straight. Distances assessed using centimeter measurements on the shaft of the instrument can be used to measure the distance of landmarks from the incisors more precisely. Circumferential extent (C value) is the depth of endoscope insertion at the GEJ to the depth of endoscope insertion from the circumferential extent of suspected columnar epithelium. While maximum extent (M value) is the depth of endoscope insertion at the GEJ to depth of endoscope insertion from the maximal extent of columnar epithelium. Endoscopic surveillance should employ four-quadrant biopsies at 2 cm intervals in patients without dysplasia and 1 cm intervals in patients with prior dysplasia. For BE patients negative for dysplasia, they should have screening endoscopy every 3-5 years.

For patients with an intermediate biopsy for dysplasia, optimal proton pump inhibitor (PPI) therapy is given for 3-6 months and then endoscopy is repeated. If the repeat endoscopy reveals the same result, then annual screening is recommended. If low-grade dysplasia is confirmed in a patient with few or no co-morbidities, endoscopic therapy with mucosal lesion resection and ablation is the preferred therapeutic choice, although annual screening is another option. Patients with BE and confirmed high-grade dysplasia should be managed with endoscopic therapy unless they have a life-limiting comorbidity.

4. Esophageal Cancer

The incidence of esophageal cancer (EC) varies depending on geographic region with Southeastern Africa and Eastern Asia showing the highest incidence and Western Africa and Central America showing lower incidence. The region from Iran through Central China, often referred to as the "esophageal cancer belt", has ninety percent of the cases of squamous cell carcinomas (SCC). Major risk factors include malnutrition, low fiber intake, and drinking hot beverages. In contrast, in areas such as the United States and several Western countries, most cases are adenocarcinoma and are attributed to cigarette use, alcohol use, and obesity. African American patients were found to have increased mortality with esophageal cancer but it is unclear whether it is an independent or dependent factor. Some studies attribute that difference to healthcare access, as evidenced by higher prevalence of Stage IV EC in African American patients, while others suggest that genetic factors might play a role in this disparity [8, 9].

The diagnosis of esophageal cancer is usually established by endoscopic biopsy. Early cancers may appear as superficial plaques, nodules, or ulcerations while advanced lesions may appear as strictures, ulcerated masses or circumferential masses. The tumor, node, metastasis (TNM) staging system of the American Joint Committee on Cancer (AJCC) and the Union for International Cancer Control (UICC) for esophageal cancer is used universally. In the most recent (eighth edition, 2017) version, tumors involving the esophagogastric junction (EGJ) with the tumor epicenter no more than 2 cm into the proximal stomach are staged as esophageal cancers. In contrast, EGJ tumors with their epicenter located more than 2 cm into the proximal stomach are staged as stomach cancers, as are all cardia cancers not involving the EGJ, even if they are within 2 cm of the EGJ. Once the diagnosis of esophageal cancer is established, pretreatment staging includes an evaluation for locoregional disease extent and an evaluation for distant metastases using endoscopic ultrasound (EUS), CT scan and PET scan.

Treatment usually depends on the staging of the disease and includes endoscopic resection, radiotherapy, chemotherapy, surgical and palliative management [10, 11].

5. Helicobacter Pylori Infection and Peptic Ulcer Disease

Helicobacter pylori (H. pylori) infection, the most common chronic bacterial infection in the world, is linked to peptic ulcer disease (PUD) and gastric adenocarcinoma. H. pylori are unique bacteria, ideally suited to live in the acidic environment of the human stomach: their spiral shape and multiple unipolar flagella allow them to move freely through the gastric mucous layer in a microenvironment protected from the low gastric pH [16]. H. pylori infection commonly occurs early in life, although the mode of transmission is usually unknown. Having an infected parent or sibling and a low-income household are both considered risk factors. In North America, the prevalence of H. pylori is related to race and socioeconomic status [20-22]. A lower prevalence is seen among Caucasians as compared to African Americans, Hispanic Americans, and Native Americans [19, 20, 23]. It is also interesting to note that African Americans with a stronger African ancestry have higher infection rates when compared to other groups which suggests a genetic predisposition to H. pylori infection [21].

Patients with peptic ulcer disease, low grade gastric mucosa associated lymphoid tissue (MALT) or a history of gastric cancer should be tested and treated. Previous antibiotic exposure and local antibiotic resistance rates should be taken into account when choosing the treatment regimen which involves antibiotics and a proton pump inhibitor (PPI) [24]. Proof of eradication is required following treatment by performing urea breath test or stool antigen testing 2-4 weeks after withholding PPI which can interfere with the results [24].

6. Gastric Cancer

Gastric cancer is the fifth most commonly diagnosed cancer worldwide [26]. Out of 22,220 cases diagnosed annually in the United States, about half are fatal [27]. There is great geographic variation in gastric cancer incidence, with the highest incidence rates in the Far East. Eastern Europe and Central and South America also have high incidence rates, while the lowest incidence rates observed in North America, North Africa, and South Asia [28]. In the United States, the incidence of gastric cancer is lower in Caucasians than it is in African Americans, Native Americans, and Hispanics. In contrast to the pattern seen with gastric non-cardia cancers, the incidence rates of gastric cardia cancer are rising [29]. The most common symptoms of gastric cancer are abdominal pain and unexplained weight loss [30]. Although the diagnosis of gastric cancer may be suspected because of findings on upper endoscopy or radiographic studies such as abdominal CT scan or barium studies, biopsy is required for definitive diagnosis. The most commonly used staging schema for gastric cancer is that of the American Joint Committee on Cancer (AJCC)/Union for International Cancer Control (UICC), which is based on TNM classifications [31]. Patients with documented gastric cancer should undergo complete staging evaluation prior to surgical exploration to help guide therapy and more reliably predict outcome. Careful staging allows the clinician to select the most appropriate therapeutic approach, minimizes unnecessary surgery, and maximizes the likelihood of benefit from the selected treatment. Treatment usually relies on a combination of surgery, chemotherapy and radiotherapy depending on the stage of the disease.

7. Acute Pancreatitis

The reported annual incidence of acute pancreatitis in the United States ranges from 5 to 35 per 100,000 population with an increase due to the rising rates of obesity and gallstones [32-33]. Smoking may increase the risk for non-gallstone-related pancreatitis by mechanisms that are unclear and may potentiate alcohol-induced damage to the pancreas [34-37]. Several studies have shown racial differences between the hospitalization rates based on race with African Americans about twice as likely to be admitted for acute pancreatitis [38-39]. There is also a difference in the underlying etiology of pancreatitis with alcoholic pancreatitis more common in African Americans. This means either greater prevalence or more genetic susceptibility in African American patients. Interestingly, African American patients also have the highest incidence of idiopathic pancreatitis.

Classically, acute pancreatitis presents with severe acute abdominal pain in the left upper quadrant with radiation to the back [14]. The occurrence of two of the following three criteria is sufficient for diagnosis: characteristic abdominal pain, elevation of serum lipase at least three times the upper limit of normal, and characteristic findings of acute pancreatitis on imaging [40, 41]. If the first two criteria are met, then imaging is not necessary for diagnosis. The severity of acute pancreatitis can be assessed clinically and using laboratory markers for fluid loss and end organ failure. There are several scores to help with this assessment including Ranson's Criteria and the bedside index for severity of acute pancreatitis (BISAP).

The cornerstone of treatment is pain and nausea control, as well as intravenous fluid hydration for correction of metabolic abnormalities. Most patients with mild pancreatitis need no further therapy and recover within several days. Patients with moderate and severe pancreatitis might require more intensive follow up especially if end organ failures develop [40, 42]. Patients with moderate or severe pancreatitis and signs of sepsis within 72 hours should be assessed for pancreatic necrosis using CT with contrast [42 , 43]. In cases where there is no response to antibiotics or in patients who are critically ill, pancreatic debridement may be necessary [44, 45]. In patients with severe pancreatitis and a prolonged inability to tolerate oral feeding, enteral nutrition is preferred over total parenteral nutrition (TPN).

8. Chronic Pancreatitis

Chronic pancreatitis is defined as an inflammatory process that causes progressive and irreversible destruction of exocrine and endocrine pancreatic glands and replaces it with fibrotic tissue. Alcohol is the leading etiology in chronic pancreatitis with a strong male to female predominance

[46-49]. In contrast to the epidemiology of acute pancreatitis, chronic pancreatitis does not seem to be associated with increased hospital admissions with the aging population. In one multicenter study examining the impact of ethnicity as a risk factor for the development of chronic pancreatitis, African Americans were 2-3 times more likely than Caucasians to be hospitalized [50].

The most common symptoms of chronic pancreatitis are severe abdominal pain and pancreatic insufficiency (exocrine and endocrine) with pancreatic cancer as the most dreaded long-term complication [51]. Although alcohol abuse is the major cause of chronic pancreatitis, smoking has also been identified as an additional independent risk factor and has been shown to be associated with the progression of chronic pancreatitis [52-55]. In terms of diagnosis, the classic constellation of pancreatic calcifications, diabetes mellitus, and steatorrhea is highly suggestive of chronic pancreatitis. The diagnosis is confirmed with abdominal CT showing calcifications or more rarely, an abnormal secretin test [51, 56]. One approach to the evaluation of a patient with suspected chronic pancreatitis in which diagnosis is unclear, is to consider abdominal imaging to rule out other causes of pain such as malignancy, or complications of pancreatitis including pseudocysts [57]. In settings where magnetic resonance cholangiopancreatography (MRCP) is available, it may be the imaging test of choice, allowing for assessment for ductal changes and potentially obviating the need for an endoscopic retrograde cholangiopancreatography (ERCP) [51, 58].

The goals of treatment include pain management, correction of pancreatic insufficiency, and management of complications. Pain management should proceed in a stepwise approach with encouragement of alcohol and smoking cessation [59]. Pancreatic enzyme supplements can be used in patients with persistent pain due to exocrine insufficiency [60-62]. Analgesics with opiates and/or nonsteroidal anti-inflammatory drugs (NSAIDs) can be considered if pancreatic enzyme therapy fails to control pain. Adjuvant therapy with pregabalin can be considered in patients who have pain that is not adequately controlled with opiates and/or NSAIDs [51, 63, 64]. Dietary modification with small frequent low-fat meals can be used in patients suffering from steatorrhea despite pancreatic enzymes. During the course of chronic pancreatitis, glucose intolerance occurs due to destruction of islet cells and may lead to overt diabetes mellitus. Management consists of a trial of oral hypoglycemic agents but insulin is frequently required [51].

9. Pancreatic Cancer

Pancreatic cancer is an aggressive cancer with a high mortality rate. It is the fourth leading cause of cancer-related death in the United States, second only to colorectal cancer when looking at gastrointestinal cancers [65]. The disease is rare before the age of 45, but the incidence increases sharply thereafter. In data from the Global Burden of Disease Study, the number of cases peaked at ages 65 to 69 in men and 75 to 79 in women [65]. There was a greater predominance in males as compared to females, and in African Americans as compared to Caucasians with worse outcomes in African Americans [66-67].

The most common presenting symptoms in patients with exocrine pancreatic cancer are painless jaundice and weight loss [14]. The initial presentation of pancreatic cancer varies according to tumor location. Approximately 60-70% of exocrine pancreatic cancers are localized to the head of the pancreas, 20-25% are in the body or tail, with the remainder involving the entire organ. Compared with tumors in the body and tail of the gland, pancreatic head tumors more often present with jaundice, steatorrhea, and weight loss [14]. At times, there may be an associated migratory superficial thrombophlebitis known classically as Trousseau's syndrome [68]. Advanced disease in particular is associated with more thromboembolic events. Rarely, nonbacterial thrombotic endocarditis may occasionally be the presenting sign of a pancreatic cancer manifesting as arterial emboli [69]. All patients presenting with jaundice or epigastric pain should have an assay of serum aminotransferases, alkaline phosphatase, and bilirubin to determine if cholestasis is present. In addition, patients with epigastric pain should be evaluated for acute pancreatitis with a serum lipase [14].

For patients with jaundice, the initial imaging study is typically an abdominal US, while abdominal CT is the preferred initial imaging test in patients presenting with epigastric pain and weight loss, but without jaundice. For patients with cholestasis who have only had an abdominal ultrasound, MRCP or ERCP is indicated, depending on the individual case [14].

Cancer antigen 19-9 (CA 19-9) is a type of tumor marker associated with pancreatic cancer. The reported sensitivity and specificity rates of CA 19-9 for pancreatic cancer range from 70-92% and 68-92%, respectively [70-72]. However, sensitivity is closely related to tumor size. Biopsy, either percutaneously or endoscopically, with histologic confirmation is required to confirm a diagnosis of pancreatic cancer. However, not all patients require a preoperative biopsy, and the next step in the workup may be a staging evaluation to determine disease extent and resectability rather than biopsy [73]. Triple-phase, contrast-enhanced, helical CT or endoscopic ultrasound (EUS) is usually warranted.

Unfortunately, surgical resection is the only potentially curative treatment for pancreatic cancer. Because of advanced disease at presentation, only about 15-20% of patients are candidates for surgery, a pancreatectomy [74-75]. Routine preoperative ERCP and biliary duct stenting to relieve jaundice has not been shown to decrease postoperative morbidity and mortality, and the procedure may actually increase the likelihood of infectious complications [76]. The most common operation for pancreatic cancer is pancreaticoduodenectomy (Whipple procedure), which removes primarily the head of the pancreas en bloc with the duodenum, distal bile duct, and proximal jejunum, with a pancreaticojejunal anastomosis [14]. Neoadjuvant therapy may represent an appropriate therapeutic option for individuals with locally advanced, unresectable, or borderline resectable non-metastatic cancer. Patients with metastatic pancreatic cancer should be offered aggressive symptomatic treatment for pain and other cancer related symptoms. Referral for a palliative care consultation should be considered early in the treatment course, especially for patients with a high symptom burden [77].

10. Hereditary Hemochromatosis

Hereditary hemochromatosis (HH), one of the most common genetic disorders in the world, is a disorder in which increased intestinal iron absorption can lead to total-body iron overload. It is most commonly due to mutations in the human homeostatic iron regulator gene (HFE gene). Two of the commonly observed HFE mutations are C282Y and H63D [78-79]. HH is known to be an autosomal recessive disorder with fairly low penetrance. This means that biallelic mutations are usually required for clinical disease, but many individuals with biallelic mutations will not be affected [14]. HH was previously thought to be a rare disorder, since the diagnosis was only made in individuals who presented with severe iron overload, but it is now appreciated as one of the most common genetic disorders in Caucasians in the United States and Europe. It is less common in individuals with African or Hispanic ancestry and extremely uncommon in individuals with Asian ancestry [80].

Clinical manifestations of HH generally do not occur until after the age of 40 years in men and after menopause in women. Nonspecific symptoms such as fatigue and lethargy are common, as are symptoms attributable to iron overload in specific organs. The liver, heart, and pituitary gland are common sites of iron overload. Untreated, patients can develop cirrhosis, hepatocellular cancer (HCC), heart failure, arrhythmias, type 2 diabetes, hypogonadism, cognitive changes, arthropathy, and bronze-colored skin.

In most cases, the initial test is serum iron studies; a transferrin saturation ≥ 45% and/or a serum ferritin > 200 ng/mL (> 200 mcg/L) in men or > 150 ng/mL (> 150 mcg/L) in women is consistent with iron overload. For those with evidence of iron overload, liver function tests and HFE mutation testing are appropriate. Magnetic resonance imaging (MRI) is generally used to quantify liver and/or cardiac iron in individuals with a ferritin > 1000 ng/mL (> 1000 mcg/L). Liver biopsy is generally reserved for individuals with suspected hepatic fibrosis or cirrhosis in which diagnosis is not confirmed [81].

Phlebotomy is the main intervention to remove excess iron. The typical schedule is once weekly until the target ferritin level is reached, with modifications as needed for anemia and other factors that affect tolerance of the procedure [81-82].

11. Viral Hepatitis

11.1. Hepatitis A

Hepatitis A infection is caused by the hepatitis A virus (HAV). Humans are the only known reservoir. Usually it is a self-limiting infection with no chronic form. Less than 1% of patients develop fulminant hepatitis and long-lasting immunity is usually achieved following infection. Hepatitis A infection can also be preventable with vaccination [14]. HAV has a fecal-oral route of transmission (either via person-to-person contact or consumption of contaminated food or water) [83]. Important risk factors include age > 50 years and chronic liver disease, including cirrhosis. Disease onset is usually marked by abrupt nausea, vomiting, fever, malaise and abdominal pain [85]. Subsequently, dark urine and pale stools develop, followed by jaundice and pruritus in a majority of the cases. The preceding symptoms with an elevation of aminotransferase levels in an area with high HAV prevalence or with a history of exposure should raise the suspicion for HAV infection [86]. The diagnosis is confirmed by recognition of serum IgM anti-HAV antibodies. Serum IgM antibodies are first seen at the beginning of symptoms, reach the peak during the convalescent phase of the disease, and remain detectable for approximately three to six months [87-88]. Treatment usually consists of supportive treatment as the majority of infections are self-limiting [88].

11.2. Hepatitis B

Hepatitis B virus (HBV) infection is a global public health problem, with an estimated 248 million HBV carriers in the world, of whom roughly 600,000 die annually due to HBV-related liver disease [89]. It is estimated that approximately two billion people worldwide have evidence of past or present infection with hepatitis B virus (HBV), and 248 million individuals are chronic carriers (i.e., positive for hepatitis B surface antigen [HBsAg]) [89-90]. The National Health and Nutrition Examination Survey (NHANES) II and III revealed that the age-adjusted prevalence of chronic HBV or previous infection in African Americans was 5.5% and 4.9%, respectively; rates that did not decrease over the previous year [91]. In addition, African American patients were found to have 3.9-fold higher risk of being positive for HBV as compared to Caucasian patients [91]. Interestingly, further analysis showed that these differences persisted after correction for important risk factors including demographic, socioeconomic and behavioral factors [92]. These data imply that other factors might play a role beside socioeconomic status.

The main mode of HBV transmission depends on the geographical area. Vertical transmission is the most common in areas with higher prevalence [92-93]. In contrast, unprotected sexual intercourse and injection drug use in adults are the major routes of transmission in lower prevalence areas [94]. The majority of patients with acute HBV infection have subclinical hepatitis, while around a third will develop symptoms. Symptoms severity may increase in cases of co-infection with another type of hepatitis [95]. In rare cases, fulminant hepatitis can occur due to massive immune-mediated lysis of infected hepatocytes [96]. Most cases of HBV are asymptomatic, except for cases of decompensated cirrhosis, or have extrahepatic manifestations, and when symptoms are present they are usually nonspecific, such as fatigue. Occasionally, some patients experience exacerbations of the infection which can mimic acute hepatitis or manifest as hepatic failure [14].

Testing for HBV infection is indicated for those with signs and symptoms of acute or chronic hepatitis. The diagnosis of acute hepatitis B is based upon the detection of HBsAg and IgM anti-HBc [97]. The diagnosis of chronic HBV infection is based upon the persistence of HBsAg for more than six months. Additional tests for HBV replication – HBeAg and serum HBV DNA, should be performed to determine the potential consideration for antiviral therapy [97].

The decision to initiate treatment is primarily based upon the presence or absence of cirrhosis, the alanine aminotransferase (ALT) level, and the HBV DNA level. There are additional indications for patients with certain concurrent conditions, such as malignancy and pregnancy. Patients who are not deemed to be treatment candidates at presentation, and those who decide to defer treatment, should undergo routine monitoring of liver biochemical tests, HBV DNA, and HBeAg status since liver disease or HBV replication may become active [97].

Currently, there are two main treatment options for chronic hepatitis B patients: treatment with a nucleoside analogue (NA) or with interferon (less commonly used now) [97]. The preferred NA regimens are monotherapies with tenofovir or entecavir. Tenofovir alafenamide (25 mg daily), if available, is usually preferred over tenofovir disoproxil fumarate (300 mg daily). Special treatment considerations exist when choosing antiviral therapy for patients with decompensated cirrhosis or reduced kidney function and for women who are pregnant [97].

Patients with chronic HBV should receive counseling on ways to prevent worsening liver disease (e.g., avoiding alcohol use, hepatitis A vaccination) and to reduce transmission to others. In addition, screening for hepatocellular carcinoma is indicated for certain high-risk patients [97].

11.3. Hepatitis C

Hepatitis C virus (HCV) infection is a leading cause of chronic liver disease worldwide, with approximately 71 million individuals infected. It has a wildly variable natural history and its pathologic effect can range from mild changes of the hepatocellular structure to extensive fibrosis, cirrhosis, and HCC [98, 99]. In the NHANES III data, it was estimated that approximately 3.9 million Americans, or 1.8% of the US population, had been exposed to HCV, and 2.7 million, or 74%, are with chronic infection. The majority of the burden included patients born between 1945 and 1965 and as expected, this cohort of patients has the highest rate of HCV related complications including cirrhosis and HCC [102-103]. In Western countries, HCV is mostly acquired through intravenous drug use or blood transfusions prior to 1990. Parenteral exposure plays a more important role in other parts of the world [104].

The diagnosis of chronic HCV infection is usually made in a patient with a reactive HCV antibody test and a positive molecular test that detects the presence of HCV RNA. If the antibody test is nonreactive, then chronic HCV infection is unlikely, and there is no need for further testing. Patients who are on hemodialysis, are severely immunocompromised, or are suspected of having an acute HCV infection may not have detectable anti-HCV antibodies despite the presence of infection. In such patients, HCV RNA testing despite a nonreactive antibody test is important to exclude infection [109].

The endpoint of therapy for HCV is a sustained virologic response (SVR) defined by undetectable RNA in serum or plasma at 12-24 weeks after the end of therapy. Both SVR12 and SVR24 have been accepted as endpoints of therapy by regulators in Europe and the United States, given that their concordance is > 99% [110]. Direct acting antiviral (DAAs) based regimens must be used in HCV-infected patients without cirrhosis or with compensated (Child-Pugh A) cirrhosis, including treatment-naïve patients and previously treated patients, because of their efficacy, ease of use, and safety [109]. Because of the risk of drug-drug interactions, a thorough risk assessment prior to starting therapy and before starting other medications during treatment is required in all patients undergoing treatment with DAAs [109].

12. Nonalcoholic Fatty Liver Disease

Nonalcoholic fatty liver disease (NAFLD) is defined as the presence of hepatic steatosis with exclusion of secondary causes of steatosis. NAFLD can progress to cirrhosis and is likely responsible for many cases that were previously labelled as cryptogenic cirrhosis. NAFLD is a global disease and one of the most common liver diseases in developed countries where the major risk factors: central obesity, type 2 diabetes mellitus, dyslipidemia, and metabolic syndrome are common [111]. Most patients with NAFLD are asymptomatic, although some patients might have fatigue and upper abdominal discomfort at times [114].

The typical biochemical pattern seen with NAFLD involves mild to moderate elevations in the aspartate aminotransferase (AST) and alanine aminotransferase (ALT) with a 2-5 fold increase over baseline values. Normal aminotransferase levels do not exclude NAFLD and it is unknown what percentage of patients with NAFLD have abnormal liver enzymes [114-115]. In order to diagnose NAFLD, other etiologies of liver disease have to be excluded. A biopsy is considered gold standard.

The management of NAFLD consists of managing the underlying liver disease when present, in addition to managing the associated comorbidities like obesity and diabetes mellitus. Pioglitazone has been shown to have some benefit in patients with diabetes mellitus [118]. Although a 3%-5% loss of body weight appears to positively influence steatosis, a greater weight loss of 7%-10% is required for histopathological improvement, including fibrosis [118]. Refraining from heavy alcohol consumption is highly recommended. In some cases, vitamin E or caffeine can be of benefit as well.

13. Inflammatory Bowel Disease

Inflammatory bowel disease (IBD) which includes Crohn's disease (CD) and ulcerative colitis (UC), affects about 1.5 million patients in the United States, 2.2 million people in Europe, and half a million more worldwide [119-120]. Data on the incidence and prevalence, disease behavior, and access to medicine of IBD among non-Caucasian populations in the United States remains conflicted and insufficient. Previous studies described mostly a Caucasian population, with other racial groups being limited by small sample size, single-center studies and limited follow-up time.

The diagnosis of IBD is established based a combination of clinical presentation, physical examination, imaging studies, and endoscopic/ histologic findings.

Therapeutic regimens are based upon the severity of the disease and the extent of gastrointestinal tract involvement. These factors may vary during the disease but accurate assessment of both is crucial in determining treatment. The severity of the disease impacts the use of anti-inflammatory drugs and risk of future complications. The extent of disease is relevant in the determination of which therapy will be most efficacious, e.g., topical, or targeted therapy.

The aims of therapy include the treatment of active disease followed by maintenance of remission. Treatment should successfully suppress active inflammatory disease medically and attempt to conserve the small bowel. Surgery should be reserved for managing complications (fistulae and abscesses) as well as treating obstruction.

14. Colorectal Cancer

Colorectal cancer (CRC) is the third most commonly diagnosed cancer, excluding skin cancer, and the second most common cause of cancer death in the United States [122, 123]. Although the overall CRC mortality has decreased over time, the incidence and mortality still vary greatly by race and ethnicity [124-126]. A number of studies have suggested that the rising mortality in African-American patients with colon cancer can be linked to more advanced cancer, differences in treatment, provider characteristics, timing of screening, and posttreatment surveillance [127-134]. Although racial and ethnic differences are most likely multifactorial, it is known that access to quality care, the receipt of definitive treatment, and socioeconomic factors have played major roles [139, 140]. Some studies have suggested that racial disparities still exist, even after controlling for socioeconomic factors and for access to equitable care and treatment [141].

The diagnosis of CRC is dependent on colonoscopy with biopsy. Preoperative clinical staging is best achieved by physical examination, CT scan of the abdomen and pelvis, and chest imaging to rule out distant metastasis.

Surgical resection is the only curative modality for localized colon cancer. Endoscopic resection may be utilized instead of radical colectomy in patients with early stage disease and favorable prognosis. For patients who had potentially curative resection of a colon cancer, postoperative (adjuvant) chemotherapy with oxaliplatin eliminates residual disease and helps increase the cure rate. These benefits have been most clearly demonstrated in patients with stage III (node-positive) disease. Most patients who present with metastatic disease are not surgical candidates, and palliative chemotherapy is usually the best course of action. However, surgery may provide a potentially curative option for some patients with single lesion hepatic metastasis. An aggressive surgical approach to both the primary and the metastatic sites is warranted in such patients in conjunction with systemic chemotherapy.

REFERENCES

[1] Park, W; Vaezi, MF. Etiology and pathogenesis of achalasia: the current understanding. *American Journal of Gastroenterology*., 2005, 100(6), 1404-14.

[2] Spechler, SJ; Talley, N; Robson, K. Achalasia: Pathogenesis, clinical manifestations, and diagnosis. *UpToDate* Waltham, MA: UpToDate. 2019.

[3] Facco, M; Brun, P; Baesso, I; Costantini, M; Rizzetto, C; Berto, A; et al. T cells in the myenteric plexus of achalasia patients show a skewed TCR repertoire and react to HSV-1 antigens. *American Journal of Gastroenterology*., 2008, 103(7), 1598-609.

[4] Chedid, V; Rosenblatt, E; Gandhi, KK; Dhalla, S; Nandwani, MC; Stein, EM; et al. The Effect of Race in Patients with Achalasia Diagnosed With High-Resolution Esophageal Manometry. *The American journal of the medical sciences.*, 2018, 355(2), 126-31.

[5] Halland, M; DeVault, KR. Esophageal Motility Disorders. *Practical Gastroenterology and Hepatology Board Review Toolkit.*, 2016, 28-35.

[6] Locke, 3rd G; Talley, NJ; Fett, SL; Zinsmeister, AR; Melton, 3rd L. Prevalence and clinical spectrum of gastroesophageal reflux: a population-based study in Olmsted County, Minnesota. *Gastroenterology.*, 1997, 112(5), 1448-56.

[7] Friedenberg, FK; Makipour, K; Palit, A; Shah, S; Vanar, V; Richter, JE. Population-based assessment of heartburn in urban Black Americans. *Diseases of the Esophagus.*, 2013, 26(6), 561-9.

[8] Greenstein, AJ; Litle, VR; Swanson, SJ; Divino, CM; Packer, S; McGinn, TG; et al. Racial disparities in esophageal cancer treatment and outcomes. *Annals of surgical oncology.*, 2008, 15(3), 881-8.

[9] Taioli, E; Wolf, AS; Camacho-Rivera, M; Kaufman, A; Lee, DS; Bhora, F; et al. Racial disparities in esophageal cancer survival after surgery. *Journal of surgical oncology.*, 2016, 113(6), 659-64.

[10] Kim, TJ; Kim, HY; Lee, KW; Kim, MS. Multimodality assessment of esophageal cancer: preoperative staging and monitoring of response to therapy. *Radiographics.*, 2009, 29(2), 403-21.

[11] Cuellar, SLB; Carter, BW; Macapinlac, HA; Ajani, JA; Komaki, R; Welsh, JW; et al. Clinical staging of patients with early esophageal adenocarcinoma: does FDG-PET/CT have a role? *Journal of Thoracic Oncology.*, 2014, 9(8), 1202-6.

[12] Fujimoto, T. Infantile hypertrophic pyloric stenosis. *Pediatric Surgery: General Principles and Newborn Surgery.*, 2020, 841-53.

[13] Schechter, R; Torfs, CP; Bateson, TF. The epidemiology of infantile hypertrophic pyloric stenosis. *Paediatric and perinatal epidemiology.*, 1997, 11(4), 407-27.

[14] Feldman, M; Friedman, LS; Brandt, LJ. *Sleisenger and Fordtran's gastrointestinal and liver disease E-book: pathophysiology, diagnosis, management*: Elsevier Health Sciences, 2015.
[15] Holder-Espinasse, M; Ahmad, Z; Hamill, J; Pahari, A; Misra, D; Drake, D; et al. Familial syndromic duodenal atresia: Feingold syndrome. *European journal of pediatric surgery.*, 2004, 14(02), 112-6.
[16] Kusters, JG; van Vliet, AH; Kuipers, EJ. Pathogenesis of Helicobacter pylori infection. *Clinical microbiology reviews.*, 2006, 19(3), 449-90.
[17] Opekun, AR; Gilger, MA; Denyes, SM; Nirken, MH; Philip, SP; Osato, MS; et al. Helicobacter pylori infection in children of Texas. *Journal of pediatric gastroenterology and nutrition.*, 2000, 31(4), 405-10.
[18] Malaty, HM; El-Kasabany, A; Graham, DY; Miller, CC; Reddy, SG; Srinivasan, SR; et al. Age at acquisition of Helicobacter pylori infection: a follow-up study from infancy to adulthood. *The Lancet.*, 2002, 359(9310), 931-5.
[19] Sinha, SK; Martin, B; Gold, BD; Song, Q; Sargent, M; Bernstein, CN. The incidence of Helicobacter pylori acquisition in children of a Canadian First Nations community and the potential for parent-to-child transmission. *Helicobacter.*, 2004, 9(1), 59-68.
[20] Nguyen, T; Ramsey, D; Graham, D; Shaib, Y; Shiota, S; Velez, M; et al. The Prevalence of Helicobacter pylori remains high in African American and Hispanic Veterans. *Helicobacter.*, 2015, 20(4), 305-15.
[21] Epplein, M; Cohen, SS; Sonderman, JS; Zheng, W; Williams, SM; Blot, WJ; et al. Neighborhood socio-economic characteristics, African ancestry, and Helicobacter pylori sero-prevalence. *Cancer Causes & Control.*, 2012, 23(6), 897-906.
[22] Epplein, M; Signorello, LB; Zheng, W; Peek, RM; Michel, A; Williams, SM; et al. Race, African ancestry, and Helicobacter pylori infection in a low-income United States population. *Cancer Epidemiology and Prevention Biomarkers.*, 2011, 20(5), 826-34.
[23] Everhart, JE; Kruszon-Moran, D; Perez-Perez, GI; Tralka, TS; McQuillan, G. Seroprevalence and ethnic differences in Helicobacter

pylori infection among adults in the United States. *The Journal of infectious diseases*., 2000, 181(4), 1359-63.

[24] Chey, WD; Leontiadis, GI; Howden, CW; Moss, SF. ACG clinical guideline: treatment of Helicobacter pylori infection. *American Journal of Gastroenterology*., 2017, 112(2), 212-39.

[25] Laine, L; Jensen, DM. Management of patients with ulcer bleeding. *American Journal of Gastroenterology*., 2012, 107(3), 345-60.

[26] Jemal, A; Bray, F; Center, MM; Ferlay, J; Ward, E; Forman, D. Global cancer statistics. *CA: a cancer journal for clinicians*., 2011, 61(2), 69-90.

[27] Siegel, R; DeSantis, C; Jemal, A. Colorectal cancer statistics, 2014. *CA: a cancer journal for clinicians*., 2014, 64(2), 104-17.

[28] Ferlay, J; Shin, HR; Bray, F; Forman, D; Mathers, C; Parkin, DM. Estimates of worldwide burden of cancer in 2008: GLOBOCAN 2008. *International journal of cancer*., 2010, 127(12), 2893-917.

[29] Sheets, SSF. *Stomach*. National Cancer Institute., 2012.

[30] Wanebo, HJ; Kennedy, B; Chmiel, J; Steele, Jr. G; Winchester, D; Osteen, R. Cancer of the stomach. A patient care study by the American College of Surgeons. *Annals of surgery*., 1993, 218(5), 583.

[31] Amin, MB; Edge, SB. *AJCC cancer staging manual*: springer, 2017.

[32] Vege, S; Yadav, D; Chari, S. Pancreatitis. *GI Epidemiology*, Talley NJ, Locke GR, Saito YA. Blackwell Publishing, Malden, MA, 2007.

[33] Toouli, J; Brooke-Smith, M; Bassi, C; Carr-Locke, D; Telford, J; Freeny, P; et al. Guidelines for the management of acute pancreatitis. *Journal of gastroenterology and hepatology*., 2002, 17, S15-S39.

[34] Lindkvist, B; Appelros, S; Manjer, J; Berglund, G; Borgström, A. A prospective cohort study of smoking in acute pancreatitis. *Pancreatology*., 2008, 8(1), 63-70.

[35] Tolstrup, JS; Kristiansen, L; Becker, U; Grønbæk, M. Smoking and risk of acute and chronic pancreatitis among women and men: a population-based cohort study. *Archives of internal medicine*., 2009, 169(6), 603-9.

[36] Yadav, D; Hawes, RH; Brand, RE; Anderson, MA; Money, ME; Banks, PA; et al. Alcohol consumption, cigarette smoking, and the risk

of recurrent acute and chronic pancreatitis. *Archives of internal medicine.*, 2009, 169(11), 1035-45.

[37] Lugea, A; Gerloff, A; Su, HY; Xu, Z; Go, A; Hu, C; et al. The combination of alcohol and cigarette smoke induces endoplasmic reticulum stress and cell death in pancreatic acinar cells. *Gastroenterology.*, 2017, 153(6), 1674-86.

[38] Fagenholz, PJ; Fernández-Del Castillo, C; Harris, NS; Pelletier, AJ; Camargo, Jr CA. Increasing United States hospital admissions for acute pancreatitis, 1988–2003. *Annals of epidemiology.*, 2007, 17(7), 491. e1-. e8.

[39] Frey, CF; Zhou, H; Harvey, DJ; White, RH. The incidence and case-fatality rates of acute biliary, alcoholic, and idiopathic pancreatitis in California, 1994-2001. *Pancreas.*, 2006, 33(4), 336-44.

[40] Tenner, S; Baillie, J; DeWitt, J; Vege, SS. American College of Gastroenterology guideline: management of acute pancreatitis. *American Journal of Gastroenterology.*, 2013, 108(9), 1400-15.

[41] Banks, PA; Bollen, TL; Dervenis, C; Gooszen, HG; Johnson, CD; Sarr, MG; et al. Classification of acute pancreatitis—2012: revision of the Atlanta classification and definitions by international consensus. *Gut.*, 2013, 62(1), 102-11.

[42] Besselink, M; van Santvoort, H; Freeman, M; Gardner, T; Mayerle, J; Vege, SS; et al. IAP/APA evidence-based guidelines for the management of acute pancreatitis. *Pancreatology.*, 2013, 13(4, suppl 2), E1-E15.

[43] Banks, PA; Freeman, ML. Gastroenterology PPCotACo. Practice guidelines in acute pancreatitis. *American journal of gastroenterology.*, 2006, 101(10), 2379-400.

[44] Yasuda, T; Ueda, T; Takeyama, Y; Shinzeki, M; Sawa, H; Nakajima, T; et al. Treatment strategy against infection: clinical outcome of continuous regional arterial infusion, enteral nutrition, and surgery in severe acute pancreatitis. *Journal of gastroenterology.*, 2007, 42(8), 681-9.

[45] Beger, HG; Bittner, R; Block, S; Büchler, M. Bacterial contamination of pancreatic necrosis: a prospective clinical study. *Gastroenterology.*, 1986, 91(2), 433-8.

[46] Spanier, BM; Dijkgraaf, MG; Bruno, MJ. Epidemiology, aetiology and outcome of acute and chronic pancreatitis: An update. *Best practice & research Clinical gastroenterology.*, 2008, 22(1), 45-63.

[47] Lankisch, P; Assmus, C; Maisonneuve, P; Lowenfels, A. Epidemiology of pancreatic diseases in Lüneburg County. *Pancreatology.*, 2002, 2(5), 469-77.

[48] Tinto, A; Lloyd, D; Kang, JY; Majeed, A; Ellis, C; Williamson, R; et al. Acute and chronic pancreatitis—diseases on the rise: a study of hospital admissions in England 1989/90-1999/2000. *Alimentary pharmacology & therapeutics.*, 2002, 16(12), 2097-105.

[49] Lowenfels, AB; Maisonneuve, P; Grover, H; Gerber, E; Korsten, MA; Antunes, MT; et al. Racial factors and the risk of chronic pancreatitis. *The American journal of gastroenterology.*, 1999, 94(3), 790-4.

[50] Yadav, D; Muddana, V; O'Connell, M. Hospitalizations for chronic pancreatitis in Allegheny County, Pennsylvania, USA. *Pancreatology.*, 2011, 11(6), 546-52.

[51] Löhr, JM; Dominguez-Munoz, E; Rosendahl, J; Besselink, M; Mayerle, J; Lerch, MM; et al. United European Gastroenterology evidence-based guidelines for the diagnosis and therapy of chronic pancreatitis (HaPanEU). *United European gastroenterology journal.*, 2017, 5(2), 153-99.

[52] Chowdhury, P; Rayford, PL. Smoking and pancreatic disorders. *European journal of gastroenterology & hepatology.*, 2000, 12(8), 869-77.

[53] Talamini, G; Bassi, C; Falconi, M; Sartori, N; Salvia, R; Rigo, L; et al. Alcohol and smoking as risk factors in chronic pancreatitis and pancreatic cancer. *Digestive diseases and sciences.*, 1999, 44(7), 1303-11.

[54] Maisonneuve, P; Lowenfels, A; Müllhaupt, B; Cavallini, G; Lankisch, P; Andersen, J; et al. Cigarette smoking accelerates progression of alcoholic chronic pancreatitis. *Gut.*, 2005, 54(4), 510-4.

[55] Maisonneuve, P; Frulloni, L; Müllhaupt, B; Faitini, K; Cavallini, G; Lowenfels, AB; et al. Impact of smoking on patients with idiopathic chronic pancreatitis. *Pancreas.*, 2006, 33(2), 163-8.

[56] Conwell, DL; Lee, LS; Yadav, D; Longnecker, DS; Miller, FH; Mortele, KJ; et al. American Pancreatic Association Practice Guidelines in Chronic Pancreatitis: evidence-based report on diagnostic guidelines. *Pancreas.*, 2014, 43(8), 1143.

[57] Luetmer, PH; Stephens, DH; Ward, EM. Chronic pancreatitis: reassessment with current CT. *Radiology.*, 1989, 171(2), 353-7.

[58] Bozkurt, T; Braun, U; Leferink, S; Gilly, G; Lux, G. Comparison of pancreatic morphology and exocrine functional impairment in patients with chronic pancreatitis. *Gut.*, 1994, 35(8), 1132-6.

[59] Whitcomb, DC; Yadav, D; Adam, S; Hawes, RH; Brand, RE; Anderson, MA; et al. Multicenter approach to recurrent acute and chronic pancreatitis in the United States: the North American Pancreatitis Study 2 (NAPS2). *Pancreatology.*, 2008, 8(4-5), 520-31.

[60] Slaff, J; Jacobson, D; Tillman, CR; Curington, C; Toskes, P. Protease-specific suppression of pancreatic exocrine secretion. *Gastroenterology.*, 1984, 87(1), 44-52.

[61] Isaksson, G; Ihse, I. Pain reduction by an oral pancreatic enzyme preparation in chronic pancreatitis. *Digestive diseases and sciences.*, 1983, 28(2), 97-102.

[62] Brown, A; Hughes, M; Tenner, S; Banks, PA. Does pancreatic enzyme supplementation reduce pain in patients with chronic pancreatitis: a meta-analysis? *American Journal of Gastroenterology.*, 1997, 92(11), 2032-5.

[63] Gilron, I; Bailey, JM; Tu, D; Holden, RR; Jackson, AC; Houlden, RL. Nortriptyline and gabapentin, alone and in combination for neuropathic pain: a double-blind, randomised controlled crossover trial. *The Lancet.*, 2009, 374(9697), 1252-61.

[64] Fioramonti, J; Bueno, L. Centrally acting agents and visceral sensitivity. *Gut.*, 2002, 51(suppl 1), i91-i5.

[65] Pourshams, A; Sepanlou, SG; Ikuta, KS; Bisignano, C; Safiri, S; Roshandel, G; et al. The global, regional, and national burden of

pancreatic cancer and its attributable risk factors in 195 countries and territories, 1990–2017: a systematic analysis for the Global Burden of Disease Study 2017. *The Lancet Gastroenterology & Hepatology.*, 2019, 4(12), 934-47.

[66] Fernandez-del Castillo, C; Jimenez, RE. *Epidemiology and nonfamilial risk factors for exocrine pancreatic cancer.* Diane MF Savarese (Ed), 105, 108, 2017, 115.

[67] Khawja, SN; Mohammed, S; Silberfein, EJ; Musher, BL; Fisher, WE; George Van Buren, I. Pancreatic cancer disparities in African Americans. *Pancreas.*, 2015, 44(4), 522-7.

[68] Khorana, AA; Fine, RL. Pancreatic cancer and thromboembolic disease. *The lancet oncology.*, 2004, 5(11), 655-63.

[69] Chen, L; Li, Y; Gebre, W; Lin, JH. Myocardial and cerebral infarction due to nonbacterial thrombotic endocarditis as an initial presentation of pancreatic adenocarcinoma. *Archives of pathology & laboratory medicine.*, 2004, 128(11), 1307-8.

[70] Pleskow, DK; Berger, HJ; Gyves, J; Allen, E; McLean, A; Podolsky, DK. Evaluation of a serologic marker, CA19-9, in the diagnosis of pancreatic cancer. *Annals of internal medicine.*, 1989, 110(9), 704-9.

[71] Ćwik, G; Wallner, G; Skoczylas, T; Ciechański, A; Zinkiewicz, K. Cancer antigens 19-9 and 125 in the differential diagnosis of pancreatic mass lesions. *Archives of surgery.*, 2006, 141(10), 968-73.

[72] DiMagno, EP; Reber, HA; Tempero, MA. AGA technical review on the epidemiology, diagnosis, and treatment of pancreatic ductal adenocarcinoma. *Gastroenterology.*, 1999, 117(6), 1464-84.

[73] Fernandez-del Castillo, C; Howell, DA; Robson, KM. Clinical manifestations, diagnosis, and staging of exocrine pancreatic cancer. *UpToDate* [online series] Waltham, MA: UpToDate. 2013.

[74] Evans, DB; Erickson, BA; Ritch, P. Borderline resectable pancreatic cancer: definitions and the importance of multimodality therapy. *Annals of surgical oncology.*, 2010, 17(11), 2803-5.

[75] Muniraj, T; Barve, P. Laparoscopic staging and surgical treatment of pancreatic cancer. *North American journal of medical sciences.*, 2013, 5(1), 1.

[76] Sohnm TA; Yeo, CJ; Cameron, JL; Pitt, HA; Lillemoe, KD. Do preoperative biliary stents increase postpancreaticoduodenectomy complications? *Journal of Gastrointestinal Surgery.*, 2000, 4(3), 258-68.

[77] Sohal, DP; Mangu, PB; Khorana, AA; Shah, MA; Philip, PA; O'Reilly, EM; et al. Metastatic pancreatic cancer: American Society of Clinical Oncology clinical practice guideline. *Journal of Clinical Oncology.*, 2016, 34(23), 2784.

[78] Feder, J; Gnirke, A; Thomas, W; Tsuchihashi, Z; Ruddy, D; Basava, A; et al. A novel MHC class I–like gene is mutated in patients with hereditary haemochromatosis. *Nature genetics.*, 1996, 13(4), 399-408.

[79] McLaren, GD; Gordeuk, VR. Hereditary hemochromatosis: insights from the hemochromatosis and iron overload screening (HEIRS) study. *ASH Education Program Book.*, 2009, 2009(1), 195-206.

[80] Crownover, BK; Covey, CJ. Hereditary hemochromatosis. *American family physician.*, 2013, 87(3), 183-90.

[81] Liver EAFTSOT. EASL clinical practice guidelines for HFE hemochromatosis. *Journal of hepatology.*, 2010, 53(1), 3-22.

[82] Bomford, A; Williams, R. Long term results of venesection therapy in idiopathic haemochromatosis. *QJM: An International Journal of Medicine.*, 1976, 45(4), 611-23.

[83] Rezende, G; Roque-Afonso, AM; Samuel, D; Gigou, M; Nicand, E; Ferre, V; et al. Viral and clinical factors associated with the fulminant course of hepatitis A infection. *Hepatology.*, 2003, 38(3), 613-8.

[84] Foster, MA; Hofmeister, MG; Kupronis, BA; Lin, Y; Xia, GL; Yin, S; et al. Increase in hepatitis A virus infections—United States, 2013–2018. *Morbidity and Mortality Weekly Report.*, 2019, 68(18), 413.

[85] Lednar, WM; Lemon, SM; Kirkpatrick, JW; Redfield, RR; Fields, ML; Kelley, PW. Frequency of illness associated with epidemic hepatitis A virus infections in adults. *American journal of epidemiology.*, 1985, 122(2), 226-33.

[86] Lai, M; Chopra, S. Hepatitis A virus infection in adults, *Epidemiology, clinical manifestations, and diagnosis.* Available at https://www.uptodate.com/contents/hepatitis-a-virus-infection-in-

adults-epidemiology-clinical-manifestations-and-diagnosis. Accessed on December 31, 2020.

[87] Wilkins, T; Malcolm, JK; Raina, D; Schade, RR. Hepatitis C: diagnosis and treatment. *American family physician.*, 2010, 81(11), 1351-7.

[88] Koff, RS. Clinical manifestations and diagnosis of hepatitis A virus infection. *Vaccine.*, 1992, 10, S15-S7.

[89] Ott, J; Stevens, G; Groeger, J; Wiersma, S. Global epidemiology of hepatitis B virus infection: new estimates of age-specific HBsAg seroprevalence and endemicity. *Vaccine.*, 2012, 30(12), 2212-9.

[90] Schweitzer, A; Horn, J; Mikolajczyk, RT; Krause, G; Ott, JJ. Estimations of worldwide prevalence of chronic hepatitis B virus infection: a systematic review of data published between 1965 and 2013. *The Lancet.*, 2015, 386(10003), 1546-55.

[91] McQuillan, GM; Coleman, PJ; Kruszon-Moran, D; Moyer, LA; Lambert, SB; Margolis, HS. Prevalence of hepatitis B virus infection in the United States: the National Health and Nutrition Examination Surveys, 1976 through 1994. *Am J Public Health.*, 1999 Jan, 89(1), 14-8.

[92] McQuillan, GM; Kruszon-Moran, D; Kottiri, BJ; Curtin, LR; Lucas, JW; Kington, RS. Racial and ethnic differences in the seroprevalence of 6 infectious diseases in the United States: data from NHANES III, 1988–1994. *American Journal of Public Health.*, 2004, 94(11), 1952-8.

[93] Beasley, R; Hwang, LY; Lin, CC; Leu, ML; Stevens, C; Szmuness, W; et al. Incidence of hepatitis B virus infections in preschool children in Taiwan. *The Journal of infectious diseases.*, 1982, 146(2), 198-204.

[94] Kim, W; Ishitani, M; Dickson, E; editors. Rising burden of Hepatitis B in the United States should 'the other' virus be forgotten? *Hepatology*; 2002: WB Saunders Co Independence Square West Curtis Center, Ste 300, Philadelphia ….

[95] Liaw, YF; Tsai, SL; Sheen, IS; Chato, M; Yeh, CT; Hsieh, SY; et al. Clinical and virological course of chronic hepatitis B virus infection

with hepatitis C and D virus markers. *The American journal of gastroenterology.*, 1998, 93(3), 354-9.

[96] Wright, TL; Mamish, D; Combs, C; Kim, M; Lake, J; Donegan, E; et al. Hepatitis B virus and apparent fulminant non-A, non-B hepatitis. *The Lancet.*, 1992, 339(8799), 952-5.

[97] Liver EAFTSOT. EASL 2017 Clinical Practice Guidelines on the management of hepatitis B virus infection. *Journal of hepatology.*, 2017, 67(2), 370-98.

[98] Blach, S; Zeuzem, S; Manns, M; Altraif, I; Duberg, AS; Muljono, DH; et al. Global prevalence and genotype distribution of hepatitis C virus infection in 2015: a modelling study. *The lancet Gastroenterology & hepatology.*, 2017, 2(3), 161-76.

[99] Razavi, H; Robbins, S; Zeuzem, S; Negro, F; Buti, M; Duberg, AS; et al. Hepatitis C virus prevalence and level of intervention required to achieve the WHO targets for elimination in the European Union by 2030: a modelling study. *The lancet Gastroenterology & hepatology.*, 2017, 2(5), 325-36.

[100] Kelen, GD; Green, GB; Purcell, RH; Chan, DW; Qaqish, BF; Sivertson, KT; et al. Hepatitis B and hepatitis C in emergency department patients. *New England Journal of Medicine.*, 1992, 326(21), 1399-404.

[101] Seeff, LB; Miller, RN; Rabkin, CS; Buskell-Bales, Z; Straley-Eason, KD; Smoak, BL; et al. 45-year follow-up of hepatitis C virus infection in healthy young adults. *Annals of internal medicine.*, 2000, 132(2), 105-11.

[102] Pyrsopoulos, N; Jeffers, L. Hepatitis C in African Americans. *Journal of clinical gastroenterology.*, 2007, 41(2), 185-93.

[103] Armstrong, GL; Wasley, A; Simard, EP; McQuillan, GM; Kuhnert WL; Alter, MJ. The prevalence of hepatitis C virus infection in the United States, 1999 through 2002. *Annals of internal medicine.*, 2006, 144(10), 705-14.

[104] Frank, C; Mohamed, MK; Strickland, GT; Lavanchy, D; Arthur, RR; Magder, LS; et al. The role of parenteral antischistosomal therapy in

the spread of hepatitis C virus in Egypt. *The Lancet.*, 2000, 355(9207), 887-91.

[105] Wiley, TE; Brown, J; Chan, J. Hepatitis C infection in African Americans: its natural history and histological progression. *The American journal of gastroenterology.*, 2002, 97(3), 700-6.

[106] Crosse, K; Umeadi, OG; Anania, FA; Laurin, J; Papadimitriou, J; Drachenberg, C; et al. Racial differences in liver inflammation and fibrosis related to chronic hepatitis C. *Clinical Gastroenterology and Hepatology.*, 2004, 2(6), 463-8.

[107] Reddy, KR; Hoofnagle, JH; Tong, MJ; Lee, WM; Pockros, P; Heathcote, EJ; et al. Racial differences in responses to therapy with interferon in chronic hepatitis C. *Hepatology.*, 1999, 30(3), 787-93.

[108] Terrault, NA; Im, K; Boylan, R; Bacchetti, P; Kleiner, DE; Fontana, RJ; et al. Fibrosis progression in African Americans and Caucasian Americans with chronic hepatitis C. *Clinical Gastroenterology and Hepatology.*, 2008, 6(12), 1403-11.

[109] European Association for the Study of the Liver. Electronic address: easloffice@easloffice.eu; European Association for the Study of the Liver. EASL Recommendations on Treatment of Hepatitis C 2018. *J Hepatol.*, 2018 Aug, 69(2), 461-511.

[110] Martinot-Peignoux, M; Stern, C; Maylin, S; Ripault, MP; Boyer, N; Leclere, L; et al. Twelve weeks posttreatment follow-up is as relevant as 24 weeks to determine the sustained virologic response in patients with hepatitis C virus receiving pegylated interferon and ribavirin. *Hepatology.*, 2010, 51(4), 1122-6.

[111] Marchesini, G; Brizi, M; Morselli-Labate, AM; Bianchi, G; Bugianesi, E; McCullough, AJ; et al. Association of nonalcoholic fatty liver disease with insulin resistance. *The American journal of medicine.*, 1999, 107(5), 450-5.

[112] Browning, JD; Kumar, KS; Saboorian, MH; Thiele, DL. Ethnic differences in the prevalence of cryptogenic cirrhosis. *LWW*, 2004.

[113] Bril, F; Portillo-Sanchez, P; Liu, IC; Kalavalapalli, S; Dayton, K; Cusi, K. Clinical and histologic characterization of nonalcoholic

steatohepatitis in African American patients. *Diabetes Care.*, 2018, 41(1), 187-92.

[114] Bacon, BR; Farahvash, MJ; Janney, CG; Neuschwander-Tetri, BA. Nonalcoholic steatohepatitis: an expanded clinical entity. *Gastroenterology.*, 1994, 107(4), 1103-9.

[115] Charatcharoenwitthaya, P; Lindor, KD; Angulo, P. The spontaneous course of liver enzymes and its correlation in nonalcoholic fatty liver disease. *Digestive diseases and sciences.*, 2012, 57(7), 1925-31.

[116] Falck-Ytter, Y; Younossi, ZM; Marchesini, G; McCullough, AJ. Clinical features and natural history of nonalcoholic steatosis syndromes. *Semin Liver Dis.*, 2001, 21(1), 17-26.

[117] McCullough, AJ. The clinical features, diagnosis and natural history of nonalcoholic fatty liver disease. *Clinics in liver disease.*, 2004, 8(3), 521-33.

[118] Chalasani, N; Younossi, Z; Lavine, JE; Charlton, M; Cusi, K; Rinella, M; et al. The diagnosis and management of nonalcoholic fatty liver disease: practice guidance from the American Association for the Study of Liver Diseases. *Hepatology.*, 2018, 67(1), 328-57.

[119] Molodecky, NA; Soon, S; Rabi, DM; Ghali, WA; Ferris, M; Chernoff, G; et al. Increasing incidence and prevalence of the inflammatory bowel diseases with time, based on systematic review. *Gastroenterology.*, 2012, 142(1), 46-54. e42.

[120] Cosnes, J; Gower–Rousseau, C; Seksik, P; Cortot, A. Epidemiology and natural history of inflammatory bowel diseases. *Gastroenterology.*, 2011, 140(6), 1785-94. e4.

[121] Afzali, A; Cross, RK. Racial and ethnic minorities with inflammatory bowel disease in the United States: a systematic review of disease characteristics and differences. *Inflammatory bowel diseases*. 2016, 22(8), 2023-40.

[122] Society, AC. Colorectal cancer facts and figures special edition 2005. *American Cancer Society Atlanta*, 2005.

[123] Ries, LA; Harkins, D; Krapcho, M; Mariotto, A; Miller, B; Feuer, EJ; et al. *SEER cancer statistics review*, 1975-2003, 2006.

[124] Polite, BN; Dignam, JJ; Olopade, OI. Colorectal cancer model of health disparities: understanding mortality differences in minority populations. *Journal of Clinical Oncology.*, 2006, 24(14), 2179-87.

[125] Clegg, LX; Li, FP; Hankey, BF; Chu, K; Edwards, BK. Cancer survival among US whites and minorities: a SEER (Surveillance, Epidemiology, and End Results) Program population-based study. *Archives of internal medicine.*, 2002, 162(17), 1985-93.

[126] Krieger, N; Quesenberry, C; Peng, T; Horn-Ross, P; Stewart, S; Brown, S; et al. Social class, race/ethnicity, and incidence of breast, cervix, colon, lung, and prostate cancer among Asian, Black, Hispanic, and White residents of the San Francisco Bay Area, 1988–92 (United States). *Cancer Causes & Control.*, 1999, 10(6), 525-37.

[127] Gray, KD; Ballard, BR; Washington, MK; Belue, R; Grady, WM; Chapman, WC; et al. Do adverse histopathologic findings in colorectal cancer patients explain disparate outcomes? *Journal of the National Medical Association.*, 2006, 98(3), 348.

[128] Chen, VW; Fenoglio-Preiser, CM; Wu, XC; Coates, RJ; Reynolds, P; Wickerham, DL; et al. Aggressiveness of colon carcinoma in blacks and whites. National Cancer Institute Black/White Cancer Survival Study Group. *Cancer Epidemiology and Prevention Biomarkers.* 1997, 6(12), 1087-93.

[129] Thomas, CR. Racial differences in the anatomical distribution of colon cancer. *Archives of Surgery.*, 1992, 127(10), 1241-5.

[130] Demissie, K; Oluwole, OO; Balasubramanian, BA; Osinubi, OO; August, D; Rhoads, GG. Racial differences in the treatment of colorectal cancer: a comparison of surgical and radiation therapy between Whites and Blacks. *Annals of epidemiology.*, 2004, 14(3), 215-21.

[131] Jessup, JM; Stewart, A; Greene, FL; Minsky, BD. Adjuvant chemotherapy for stage III colon cancer: implications of race/ethnicity, age, and differentiation. *Jama.*, 2005, 294(21), 2703-11.

[132] Nadel, MR; Blackman, DK; Shapiro, JA; Seeff, LC. Are people being screened for colorectal cancer as recommended? Results from the

National Health Interview Survey. *Preventive medicine.*, 2002, 35(3), 199-206.

[133] McMahon, Jr. LF; Wolfe, RA; Huang, S; Tedeschi, P; Manning, Jr. W; Edlund, MJ. Racial and gender variation in use of diagnostic colonic procedures in the Michigan Medicare population. *Medical care.*, 1999, 712-7.

[134] Gornick, ME; Eggers, PW; Riley, GF. Associations of race, education, and patterns of preventive service use with stage of cancer at time of diagnosis. *Health services research.*, 2004, 39(5), 1403-28.

[135] Baldwin, LM; Dobie, SA; Billingsley, K; Cai, Y; Wright, GE; Dominitz, JA; et al. Explaining black–white differences in receipt of recommended colon cancer treatment. *Journal of the National Cancer Institute.*, 2005, 97(16), 1211-20.

[136] Ayanian, JZ; Zaslavsky, AM; Fuchs, CS; Guadagnoli, E; Creech, CM; Cress, RD; et al. Use of adjuvant chemotherapy and radiation therapy for colorectal cancer in a population-based cohort. *Journal of clinical oncology.*, 2003, 21(7), 1293-300.

[137] Ball, JK; Elixhauser, A. Treatment differences between blacks and whites with colorectal cancer. *Medical care.*, 1996, 970-84.

[138] Shavers, VL; Brown, ML. Racial and ethnic disparities in the receipt of cancer treatment. *Journal of the National Cancer Institute.*, 2002, 94(5), 334-57.

[139] Cooper, GS; Yuan, Z; Landefeld, CS; Rimm, AA. Surgery for colorectal cancer: race-related differences in rates and survival among Medicare beneficiaries. *American journal of public health.*, 1996, 86(4), 582-6.

[140] Wegner, EL; Kolonel, LN; Nomura, AM; Lee, J. Racial and socioeconomic status differences in survival of colorectal cancer patients in Hawaii. *Cancer.*, 1982, 49(10), 2208-16.

[141] Du, XL; Fang, S; Vernon, SW; El-Serag, H; Shih, YT; Davila, J; et al. Racial disparities and socioeconomic status in association with survival in a large population-based cohort of elderly patients with colon cancer. *Cancer: Interdisciplinary International Journal of the American Cancer Society.*, 2007, 110(3), 660-9.

In: Care of the Older African Adult
Editor: Seki A. Balogun
ISBN: 978-1-53619-295-7

Chapter 12

UROGYNECOLOGIC DISEASES IN OLDER AFRICAN ADULTS

Olufemi O. Aworinde[1,*], Olufemi O. Ojewuyi[2,†] and Adetunji O. Adeniji[3,‡]

[1]Consultant Obstetrician and Gynaecologist,
Department of Obstetrics and Gynaecology,
Bowen University, Iwo, Oyo state, Nigeria
[2]Consultant Urological Surgeon,
Department of Surgery,
Osun State University Teaching Hospital,
Osogbo, Osun state, Nigeria
[3]Professor of Obstetrics and Gynecology,
Department of Obstetrics and Gynecology,
Ladoke Akintola University of Technology,
Ogbomoso, Oyo State, Nigeria

Keywords: pelvic, floor, prolapse, incontinence, prostate, enlargement, erectile, dysfunction, bladder

* Corresponding Author's E-mail: aworindeolufemi@yahoo.com.
† Corresponding Author's E-mail: phemmyoje@yahoo.com.
‡ Corresponding Author's E-mail: tunji1802@yahoo.com.

ABSTRACT

Urogynecologic diseases in older adults differ between the male and female gender due to the uniqueness of their urogenital systems. While the females have mostly pelvic floor disorders such as pelvic organ prolapse and urinary incontinence; males grapple with prostate-related issues ranging from benign to malignant.

Many of these diseases are chronic in nature and have great impact on the quality of life of the patients, as well as socioeconomic implications for patients and their family, and the society at large. Medical care in most African countries is self-funded and without medical insurance, placing significant hardship on patients and their relatives. This more often than not, also limits the options of treatment that are available to these patients.

In this chapter, we discuss the epidemiology and clinical management of common urogynecologic disorders in older African males and females.

1. PELVIC ORGAN PROLAPSE

1.1. Epidemiology

About half of all older women when examined are noted to have pelvic organ prolapse (POP) but only 3 - 6% will present with symptoms [1]. In studies on African women, the prevalence ranges from 12 to 64% [2–5]. The prevalence of pelvic organ prolapse increases with age until its peak in the seventh decade; older parous women show progressive disease and are unlikely to have regression of their prolapse [6]. Anterior compartment prolapse is the most common type of POP seen [7].

Other associated risk factors include vaginal delivery, forceps delivery, obesity, chronic cough, constipation, repeated heavy lifting and hysterectomy [6].

1.2. Clinical Presentation

Most patients with POP are asymptomatic. In those with symptoms, the feeling of a mass protruding from the vagina is the most common presentation [6]. Other possible presentations include urinary retention, vaginal discharge, sexual difficulty and feeling of incomplete bladder emptying.

A pelvic examination helps to determine the location and extent of the prolapse, including valsalva maneuver, which is often needed to determine the full extent of the prolapse [8]. The extent of the prolapse is classified using the pelvic organ prolapse quantification staging system or the Baden-Walker grading system [6].

1.3. Clinical Management

The goal of treatment is to improve symptoms and minimize prolapse progression. The options of management include conservative management, pelvic floor exercises, use of pessary and surgery [9]. Since majority of the patients with POP are asymptomatic, treatment may not be needed. In instances where the mass does not protrude beyond the hymen and does not negatively impact the quality of life, conservative management is also considered [6]. Kegel exercises (60 exercises divided into three sets per day) have been found to improve symptoms associated with incontinence and mild prolapse without treating or reversing the disease [9].

Use of pessaries can be considered for all stages of prolapse and have been found to delay both the progression of the prolapse and the need for surgical intervention [10]. Ring pessary is the most commonly used in Africa.

Obliterative and reconstructive surgeries for POP include hysterectomy and hysteropexy. The decision for surgery in older women depends on expectations for body image and desire for future vaginal intercourse [6]. In Africa, the most common surgery done for women in this age group is vaginal hysterectomy with pelvic floor repair. It gives room for sexual intercourse as well as gives a good body image based on cultural values. Other options include colpocleisis, sacrocolpopexy and transvaginal mesh. The options of management are limited by availability of surgical expertise and cost of the procedure.

2. Urinary Incontinence

2.1. Epidemiology

The prevalence of urinary incontinence (UI) varies within population and gender. It is said to be about 3 – 72%; only 25% of older adults receive treatment. Women report incontinence more often than men; the most common being stress incontinence. In men, benign prostatic hyperplasia may result in overflow incontinence and with treatment, they may develop stress incontinence [12]. Occurrence of UI is influenced by age, parity, childbirth, obesity, diuretics and medical comorbidities such as diabetes mellitus [11].

2.2. Clinical Presentation

Urinary incontinence (UI) is defined as the complaint of involuntary leakage of urine; which may be transient or chronic [11]. Depending on the aetiology and presentation, chronic UI can be classified into stress (leakage associated with episodes of increased intra-abdominal pressure), urge (leakage associated with urgency and involuntary detrusor muscle activity), overflow (leakage associated with dribbling of urine due to inability to empty the bladder), mixed (combination of stress and urge incontinence) and functional (leakage of urine due to environmental, mental or physical barriers to toileting).

A detailed history and examination would help in identifying the type of UI and this guides the management.

2.3. Clinical Management

Having ruled out transient incontinence from the history, efforts should be geared towards determining the type of chronic incontinence the patient has. Urinary incontinence questionnaire is a helpful tool in this regard. The Questionnaire for Urinary Incontinence Diagnosis (QUID) is a 6- item validated questionnaire which is used to determine if the UI is predominantly stress or urge [13]. The history should rule out medical comorbidities and determine the severity of symptoms and the effect of UI on quality of life. The latter would help guide the intensity and aggressiveness of treatment [14]. A voiding diary may come in handy if the patient provides an unclear voiding history. The physical examination should involve all systems to rule out any comorbidities. A pelvic examination is useful in both genders, to evaluate the pelvic floor in females and the prostate in males. Renal function test typically needs to be performed to exclude renal compromise from urinary retention and back pressure effects on the kidney, which may be found in overflow incontinence. Measurement of post void urine residual volume (PVR) is also very important in the diagnosis of overflow incontinence. PVR measurement less than 50mls excludes overflow incontinence [14]. More complex urodynamic studies and cystoscopy may be necessary in some instances to aid diagnosis. The criteria for when and in whom to do complex urodynamic studies is unclear and usually depends on individual expert opinions [12].

The treatment of urinary incontinence is a stepwise care plan, best tailored to the type of UI and its etiology. Conservative management, lifestyle and behavioral modifications, pelvic muscle training, adjunctive therapy, mechanical devices, pharmacologic therapy and surgery are offered sequentially [15]. Life style modification include weight control, cessation of smoking, restriction of caffeine and fluid intake, as well as treatment of constipation. Various studies have shown these steps to be helpful in some patients. Kegel exercises and pessaries just like in POP have been found to be helpful. Adjunctive therapy include vaginal cone, biofeedback, electrical stimulation and acupuncture [12].

Pharmacologic therapy have been found to be more useful in urge UI than in stress UI. They include estrogen, antimuscarinic agents, beta agonists and onabotulinumtoxinA.

Surgical options for stress incontinence involves increasing urethral outlet resistance with procedures such as bladder neck suspension, periurethral bulking therapy, mid-urethral slings, artificial urinary sphincter, transobturator male sling and transobturator vaginal tape. Surgical procedures used in treatment of urge incontinence include sacral nerve modulation and bladder augmentation which target improved bladder compliance [15].

3. Benign Prostatic Hyperplasia (BPH)

3.1. Epidemiology

Prostatic disease is generally regarded as a disease of aging and BPH is among the most common of these conditions which affect older men [16]. The reported prevalence of microscopic, macroscopic and clinical BPH varies among races. Only a few population-based studies of BPH have been conducted in Africa. In a recent study in West Africa, the prevalence of DRE-detected BPH was 62.3% in men aged 50 - 74 years, and based on PSA higher than1.5ng/ml, 58.1% in men aged 70 - 74 years. This is higher than reported in the United States, where higher prevalence was also reported in African-Americans compared to Caucasian-Americans [16].

3.2. Clinical Presentation

BPH manifests in form of lower urinary tract symptoms (LUTS). However, of importance is the fact that LUTS is not specific for BPH, other pathologies of the lower urinary tract e.g., urethral stricture, prostate cancer also present with LUTS. The internationally accepted and most often used method of evaluating patients with symptomatic BPH is the International Prostate Symptoms Score (IPSS) [17]. It is an assessment method based on self-reported LUTS and the quality of life of the patient. LUTS includes the irritative (storage) symptoms; frequency, nocturia, urgency, urge incontinence and obstructive (voiding) symptoms; hesitancy, poor urinary stream, straining, intermittency and feeling of incomplete emptying of bladder. Seven of these parameters are included in the IPSS, each with a maximum score of five. The total score is 35. Based on the IPSS, patient is categorized as having mild symptoms 0 - 7, moderate, 8 - 19 and severe symptoms 20 - 35. Digital rectal examination findings of symmetrically enlarged, smooth, firm (rubbery), and non-nodular prostate is suggestive of BPH.

3.3. Clinical Management

BPH is a diagnosis of exclusion and usually would not require histological diagnosis. Prostate specific antigen (PSA) is done and a value of 0 - 4ng/ml is considered normal, even though, there is also age-specific PSA. Transrectal ultrasound is done to evaluate the prostate volume and also its echogenicity. Prostate volume estimated from studies in Nigeria is more than that amongst Caucasians [18].

The approach to the treatment of BPH in African men is similar to what obtains in developed countries. Based on the severity of symptoms, patients are offered options of care available ranging from medical therapy to minimally invasive therapy or open surgery. Patients with mild to moderate IPSS score would usually benefit from medical therapy. Those with severe IPSS score more often than not, require surgery. Absolute indication for surgery include; failure of medical therapy, coexisting bladder stones, recurrent haematuria, recurrent urinary tract infection, chronic urinary retention, renal failure from obstructive uropathy. Open surgery is more commonly performed in Africa compared to Western nations, this is due to the dearth of expertise and the high cost of minimally invasive surgery. In addition, the relatively bigger size of the prostate in Africans is more amenable to open surgery [18].

4. EPIDIDYMORCHITIS

4.1. Epidemiology

Epididymorchitis is the inflammation of the epididymis and the testes which often result from ascending infection of the urinary tract [19]. It can also be blood-borne or occur from direct inoculation. It is one of the relatively common urological conditions seen during routine clinic visits or even sometimes in the emergency room. Though, it may be considered not to be of public health importance in terms of the epidemiology, it places a psychological burden on the patients with significant impact on the quality of life. Two peak ages have been documented with regards to the incidence of epididymorchitis; the second and the sixth decade of life [20]. In older men, bladder outlet obstruction, urethral instrumentation and urinary tract surgery are the major predisposing factors.

4.2. Clinical Presentation

Epididymorchitis can either present in form of an acute scrotum which is a urological emergency or as a chronic disease. Either form of presentation can occur at any age. The aetiopathogenesis varies depending on the age group [19]. In older African men, the common pathogen is *Escherichia coli* with the mode of infection due to ascending infection from the urethra. In the younger age group, it usually results from sexually transmitted infection, Neisseria gonorrhea and Chlamydia trachomatis are the implicated organisms and it must be clearly differentiated from testicular torsion. The acute form is characterized by fever, pain with or without swelling in the affected hemi-scrotum, and the symptom duration is usually less than 6 weeks. Older men often give history of background lower urinary tract symptoms, recent urethral instrumentation or surgery. The chronic disease form of presentation is with much less pain and swelling and usually takes a longer time to resolve. Quite a number of patients in Nigeria and most of sub-Saharan Africa present late due to the availability of many over the counter antibiotics and alternative medicine providers. They also sometimes may present with complications such as scrotal abscess that would require incision and drainage and Fournier's gangrene in extreme cases of delayed presentation.

4.3. Clinical Management

This includes laboratory testing: urinalysis, urine microscopy and culture, complete blood count, doppler scrotal ultrasound. There is presently no guideline for the treatment of epididymorchitis in Nigeria. In the United Kingdom (UK), Nicholson et al. reported that the treatment of epididymorchitis by general practitioners is not clear because guidelines are not being followed [21]. The treatment consist of bed rest, scrotal elevation, change of urethral catheter (if present) and use of parenteral antibiotics. The initial choice of antibiotics is usually empirical. Subsequent change in antibiotic choice depends on the result of urine culture and sensitivity. Fluoroquinolones is the initial choice of antibiotics in African countries, similar to the practice in the UK [21]. Non-steroidal anti-inflammatory drugs may also be useful for symptomatic relief. In situations in which patients present with scrotal abscess, incision and drainage is performed with recommended subsequent regular sitz-baths.

5. Erectile Dysfunction

5.1. Epidemiology

Erectile dysfunction is defined as the inability to achieve or sustain erection necessary for satisfactory sexual intercourse. It is the most common entity of male sexual dysfunction which also includes disorders of libido and ejaculation [22]. It is a disease of public health importance considering its increasing magnitude, association with chronic medical conditions and significant psychosocial impact [22]. The social stigma and myths associated with erectile dysfunction have made its management a more tedious experience compared to what is obtainable in developed countries. Even though the likelihood of erectile dysfunction increases with aging, it should not be regarded as an inevitable consequence of aging [22]. The psychological effects that could result include perceived unwillingness to initiate sexual relationships because of the fear of failure or rejection and this more often than not, has a negative impact on the overall quality of life especially in older men [21]. The prevalence of ED varies with age, race, ethnicity, socioeconomic and health status of affected individuals [19]. In Nigeria, the overall prevalence of ED is 43.8% [22], despite this, only a few receive medical treatment. Men of African descent have been found to have greater risk of developing ED in their lifetime than the Caucasians [23]. Reasons attributed to this include: lifestyle habits and health conditions, poor socioeconomic status, psychosocial issues, anxiety and poor partner relationships. In studies in Nigerian men, the overall prevalence of ED was higher compared to those from Asia, Europe and Canada [22].

The etiology of ED are considered to be psychogenic, organic or mixed. The psychological causes of ED includes; anxiety, depression, bereavement, marital stress, financial stress. The organic causes are more common in the older men and include; vascular causes (diabetes mellitus, hypertension, arteriosclerosis), hypogonadism, previous prostate surgery [22], chronic alcoholism which causes polyneuropathy and hypogonadism. ED is considered as a symptom of damage to the vascular endothelium [23]. Nitric oxide synthesized by the endothelium is responsible for smooth muscle relaxation with increased blood flow to the sinusoidal spaces and erection. Severe hypertension is known to result in endothelial dysfunction with consequent impaired nitric oxide production. ED has been known to occur at an earlier age in patients with diabetes than the general population and it can also be the first symptom of an underlying cardiovascular disease. Tobacco smoking is also associated with ED, smokers are approximately 1.5 times likely to report ED than non-smokers [23]. Antihypertensives; B blockers, thiazides, are also causative factor for erectile dysfunction unlike angiotensin-converting enzyme inhibitors (ACEI), angiotensin II receptor blockers (ARBs) and calcium channel blockers [22].

5.2. Clinical Management

The international index of erectile function (IIEF)-5, validated in many studies worldwide including studies in Africa [22], is the gold standard measure in assessing ED and is also used in clinical trials for assessment of treatment efficacy [23]. It has five domains; erectile function, orgasmic function, sexual desire, intercourse satisfaction and overall satisfaction. Based on the total score, patients are categorized as having mild, moderate, or severe ED. Mild ED appears to be more prevalent in studies done in Nigeria [22]. A major hindrance to the management of ED in Africa are the myth and misconceptions surrounding this condition. This includes the misconception that it is a normal part of aging, it has no impact on the partner and can be well treated with herbal supplements only. Almost 39% of Nigerian men believe ED is a myth. Less than half of Nigerian men (40.9%) discuss sex freely with anybody including their spouse and physicians. In addition, most primary care physicians in Nigeria (62%) do not ask patients about their sexual function unless they bring it up [23]. The options of treatment include: phosphodiesterase-5 inhibitor therapy, which is the first option of therapy, second option is intracavernosal injection and the third option is penile implant [24].

6. Bladder Cancer

6.1. Epidemiology

Bladder cancer is the second most common cancer of the genitourinary tract. It is considered to be of public health importance, especially in parts of Africa where schistosomiasis is still endemic. The peak age of diagnosis is 65 years of age and it is more common in males [25]. The predominant histological types are the transitional cell carcinoma (TCC) and the squamous cell carcinoma (SCC). While TCC is predominant in the developed countries [25], SCC is the most common in Africa. Though there are now increasing cases of TCC in Africa as a result of increased industrialization, overall, SCC is still the most common [26].

Exposure to industrial chemicals and smoking remains the major risk factors associated with the pathogenesis of bladder cancer in the developed world. In most parts of Africa, schistosomiasis is still the most predominant risk factor followed by smoking, exposure to dyes and industrial chemicals [25, 26]. Patients on cyclophosphamide for other malignant conditions such as breast cancer are also at risk of developing bladder cancer.

6.2. Clinical Presentation

Patients with TCC often present with painless haematuria, while in Africa with high incidence of SCC, they may present with painful haematuria, necroturia, irritative lower urinary tract symptoms and bladder mass [26]. SCC patients more often than not present with muscle-invasive disease. TCC tends to be multifocal and non-muscle invasive at presentation. This may be because the pathogenesis of schistosomiasis in the bladder starts from within the perivesical plexus which allows for disease progression from the serosa to the mucosa [27]. The reverse is the case in patients with TCC.

6.3. Clinical Management

Management of bladder cancer is based on the stage of the disease at presentation and also the histological type. Options include surgery, chemotherapy and radiotherapy. The disease classification relevant in management is based on whether it is muscle invasive or not. For muscle invasive disease, options include radical cystectomy and urinary diversion or chemoradiation for advanced disease in TCC. For SCC, it is both radio-resistant and chemo-resistant, and the only available option is often cystectomy and urinary diversion.

For non-muscle invasive disease, transurethral resection of the bladder tumour (TURBT) followed by intravesical chemotherapy/immunotherapy is usually recommended. The prognosis of TCC is overall better than SCC [27].

7. Prostate Cancer

7.1. Epidemiology

Cancer of the prostate (CaP) is the most frequently diagnosed non-cutaneous malignancy worldwide and it is the second leading cause of death in men in the Western world [28]. In the developed world, at the time of diagnosis, the disease is mostly confined to the prostate, otherwise referred to as organ-confined CaP, and only about 20% would have metastasized to other tissues [29].

Unfortunately, the reverse is the trend in developing countries where larger percentage of patients present with advanced disease [30]. The early diagnosis in the United States and most other countries in the developed world is attributed to the classification of CaP as one of the diseases of public health importance. The prevalence of CaP increases with age and continues to increase with advancing age unlike most other malignancies with peak age of incidence. The incidence of CaP varies by race and ethnicity, with the highest incidence among the African Americans and older adults of African descent. In a recent hospital based study, CaP was reported as the number one cancer in Nigerian men constituting up to 16.7% of male cancers [30].

CaP patients of African descent tend to present with higher grade disease, have higher PSA levels and have a greater incidence of metastatic disease.

7.2. Clinical Presentation

CaP may be asymptomatic. It may also present as a localized disease, locally advanced or metastatic disease. Elevated PSA detected during routine screening in the absence of symptoms and signs may be a pointer to CaP, this is categorized as T1c in the TNM staging. Localized disease is characterized by the presence of lower urinary tract symptoms (LUTS), especially irritative symptoms such as frequency, nocturia, urgency and urge incontinence. With locally advanced disease, there may be, in addition to LUTS, lower limb swelling from infiltration of the lymph nodes or features of obstructive uropathy from infiltration of the ureteric orifices.

CaP is one of the most common malignancies that metastasizes to the bone in men with consequent occurrence of skeletal-related events (SREs) such as low back pain, long bone pain, pathological fracture, and cord compression [31]. Haematogenous spread to the viscera though not as common as bone metastases, can also occur, especially when it is the aggressive type. Large intestinal obstruction due to the pressure effect of the prostatic mass protruding into the rectal lumen may also occur.

7.3. Clinical Management

The management of CaP just like most other malignancies depends on the stage of the disease; whether it is organ confined, locally advanced or metastatic disease. Important factors in grading and staging of CaP include: serum PSA, the gleason score, results of investigations such as abdominopelvic ultrasound, prostate biopsy for histology, abdominopelvic CT scan, and bone scan. For organ confined disease, options include surgery and radiotherapy. The surgical procedure most commonly done is radical retropubic prostatectomy. Approach to this surgery can be open or laparoscopic robotic. Most centers in sub-Saharan Africa perform open surgery. Localized and metastatic disease requires multimodal approach; surgery and/or radiotherapy or androgen deprivation therapy (ADT). Currently, ADT is the cornerstone of treatment of metastatic disease [32].

CaP is largely androgen-dependent and responds to endocrine therapy. ADT is an effective treatment modality in metastatic disease, it decreases the rate of disease progression, alleviates symptoms and prolongs patient survival [32].

References

[1] Barber, M. D., Maher, C. Epidemiology and outcome assessment of pelvic organ prolapse. *Int. Urogynecol. J.,* 2013 Nov.; 24(11): 1783 - 90.

[2] Masenga, G. G., Shayo, B. C., Rasch, V. Prevalence and risk factors for pelvic organ prolapse in Kilimanjaro, Tanzania: A population based study in Tanzanian rural community. *PLoS ONE,* 2018; 13(4): e0195910.

[3] Scherf, C., Morison, L., Fiander, A., Ekpo, G., Walraven, G. Epidemiology of pelvic organ prolapse in rural Gambia, West Africa. *BJOG,* 2002 Apr.; 109(4):431 - 6.

[4] Wusu-Ansah, O. K., Opare-Addo, H. S. Pelvic organ prolapse in rural Ghana. *Int. J. Gynaecol. Obstet.,* 2008 Nov.; 103(2):121 - 4.

[5] Megabiaw, B., Adefris, M., Rortveit, G., Degu, G., Muleta, M., Blystad, A., Kiserud, T., Melese, T., Kebede, Y. Pelvic floor disorders among women in Dabat district, northwest Ethiopia: A pilot study. *Int. Urogynecol. J.,* 2013 Jul.; 24(7):1135 - 43.

[6] Iglesia, C. B., Smithling, K. R. Pelvic Organ Prolapse. *Am. Fam. Physician*, 2017; 1; 96(3):179 - 185.

[7] Wu, J. M., Vaughan, C. P., Goode, P. S. et al. Prevalence and trends of symptomatic pelvic floor disorders in U.S. women. *Obstet. Gynecol.,* 2014; 123(1):141 - 148.

[8] Meyer, I., Howard, T. F., Smith, H. J., Kim, K. H., Richter, H. E. (2020). Gynecologic Disorders in the Older Woman. In: Rosenthal, R., Zenilman, M., Katlic, M. (eds) *Principles and Practice of Geriatric Surgery*. Springer, Cham.

[9] Committee on Practice Bulletins—Gynecology and the American Urogynecologic Society. Practice bulletin no. 176: pelvic organ prolapse. *Obstet. Gynecol.,* 2017; 129(4):e56 - e72.

[10] Jones, K. A., Harmanli, O. Pessary use in pelvic organ prolapse and urinary incontinence. *Rev. Obstet. Gynecol.,* 2010; 3(1):3 - 9.

[11] Ojengbede, O. A., Morhason-Bello, I. O., Adedokun, B. O., Okonkwo, N. S., Kolade, C. O. Prevalence and the associated trigger factors of urinary incontinence among 5000 black women in sub-Saharan Africa: Findings from a community survey. *BJU Int.,* 2011; 107(11):1793 - 800.

[12] Hu, J. S., Pierre, E. F. Urinary Incontinence in Women: Evaluation and Management. *Am. Fam. Physician,* 2019; 100(6):339 - 348. PMID: 31524367.

[13] Bradley, C. S., Rahn, D. D., Nygaard, I. E., Barber, M. D., Nager, C. W., Kenton, K. S. et al. The questionnaire for urinary incontinence diagnosis (QUID): Validity and responsiveness to change in women undergoing non-surgical therapies for treatment of stress predominant urinary incontinence. *Neurourol. Urodyn.,* 2010; 29(5): 727 - 734.

[14] Khandelwal, C., Kistler, C. Diagnosis of urinary incontinence. *Am. Fam. Physician,* 2013; 15; 87(8):543 - 50. PMID: 23668444.

[15] Committee on Practice Bulletins—Gynecology and the American Urogynecologic Society. ACOG Practice Bulletin No. 155: Urinary Incontinence in Women. *Obstet. Gynecol.,* 2015; 126(5):e66 - 81.

[16] Chokkalingam, A. P., Yeboah, E. D., Demarzo, A., Netto, G., Yu, K., Biritwum, R. B. et al. Prevalence of BPH and lower urinary tract symptoms in West Africans. *Prostate Cancer and Prostatic Diseases,* 2012; 15(2):170 - 176.

[17] Barry, M. J., Fowler, F. J., Jr., O'Leary, M. P., Bruskewitz, R. C., Holtgrewe, H. L., Mebust, W. K. et al. The American Urological Association symptom index for benign prostatic hyperplasia. The Measurement Committee of the American Urological Association. *The Journal of Urology,* 1992; 148(5):1549 - 1557.

[18] Mohammed, A., Bello, A., Maitama, H., Ajibola, H., Lawal, A., Isah, M. et al. Determination of prostatic volume and characteristics by

transrectal ultrasound among patients with lower urinary tract symptoms in Zaria, Nigeria. *Archives of International Surgery,* 2014; 4(1):31 - 35.

[19] Banyra, O., Shulyak, A. Acute epididymo-orchitis: Staging and treatment. *Central European Journal of Urology*, 2012; 65(3):139.

[20] Redshaw, J. D., Tran, T. L., Wallis, M. C., deVries, C. R. Epididymitis: A 21-year retrospective review of presentations to an outpatient urology clinic. *The Journal of urology,* 2014; 192(4):1203 - 1207.

[21] Nicholson, A., Rait, G., Murray-Thomas, T., Hughes, G., Mercer, C. H., Cassell, J. Management of epididymo-orchitis in primary care: results from a large UK primary care database. *British Journal of General Practice,* 2010; 60(579):e407 - e422.

[22] Adebusoye, L. A., Olapade-olaopa, O. E., Ladipo, M. M., Owoaje, E. T. Prevalence and correlates of erectile dysfunction among primary care clinic attendees in Nigeria. *Global Journal of Health Science,* 2012; 4(4):107.

[23] Yovwin, D., Imarhiagbe, F., Obazee, E., Oguike, T. Erectile dysfunction in a sub-saharan African population: Profile and correlates in a tertiary care hospital. *Sahel Medical Journal,* 2015; 18(3):116 - 120.

[24] Mobley, D. F., Khera, M., Baum, N. Recent advances in the treatment of erectile dysfunction, *Postgraduate Medical Journal,* 2017; 93:679 - 685.

[25] Chavan, S., Bray, F., Lortet-Tieulent, J., Goodman, M., Jemal, A. International variations in bladder cancer incidence and mortality. *European urology,* 2014; 66(1):59 - 73.

[26] Zaghloul, M. S. Bladder cancer and schistosomiasis. *Journal of the Egyptian National Cancer Institute*, 2012; 24(4):151 - 159.

[27] Martin, J. W., Carballido, E. M., Ahmed, A., Farhan, B., Dutta, R., Smith, C. et al. Squamous cell carcinoma of the urinary bladder: Systematic review of clinical characteristics and therapeutic approaches. *Arab journal of urology*, 2016; 14(3):183 - 191.

[28] Siegel, R., Ward, E., Brawley, O., Jemal, A. Cancer statistics, 2011. *CA: A Cancer Journal for Clinicians*, 2011; 61(4):212 - 236.

[29] Altekruse, S., Kosary, C., Krapcho, M., Neyman, N., Aminou, R., Waldron, W. et al. *SEER Cancer Statistics Review*, 1975 - 2007: National Cancer Institute. Bethesda, MD, based on November 2009 SEER data submission, posted to the SEER web site, 2010. seer cancer gov/csr. 2011.

[30] Ojewuyi, O. O., Ikuerowo, S. O., Jeje, E. A., Adewole, O. A., Abolarinwa, A. A., Omisanjo, O. A. Bone mineral density in Nigerian men on androgen deprivation therapy for advanced prostate cancer. *African Journal of Urology*, 2020; 26(1):1 - 6.

[31] Cathomas, R., Bajory, Z., Bouzid, M., El Ghoneimy, A., Gillessen, S., Goncalves, F. et al. Management of bone metastases in patients with castration-resistant prostate cancer. *Urologia internationalis,* 2014; 92(4):377 - 386.

[32] Chen, C. H., Hsieh, J. T., Huang, K. H., Pu. Y. S., Chang, H. C. Predictive clinical indicators of biochemical progression in advanced prostate cancer patients receiving Leuplin depot as androgen deprivation therapy. *PLoS One,* 2014 Aug. 14; 9(8):e105091.

LIST OF CONTRIBUTORS

(in alphabetical order)

Emaad Abdel Rahman, MD, PhD, FASN.
Professor of Internal Medicine, Division of Nephrology, University of Virginia Health System, Charlottesville, Virginia, United States.

Oluyemisi Abdulsalam, MD, FACE, FACP
Clinical Endocrinologist, Veterans Affairs Medical Center, Fayetteville, North Carolina

Adetunji O. Adeniji, MBBS, FWACS, FMCOG
Professor of Obstetrics and Gynecology, Department of Obstetrics and Gynecology, Ladoke Akintola University of Technology, Ogbomoso, Oyo State, Nigeria

Mohamed Ahmed, MD
Resident physician, Department of Internal Medicine, University of Missouri- Kansas city, Missouri, United States.

Olufemi Aworinde, MBBS, FWACS, FMCOG
Consultant Obstetrician and Gynecologist, Department of Obstetrics and Gynecology, Bowen University, Iwo, Oyo state, Nigeria.

Seki A. Balogun, MBBS, FACP, AGSF
Associate Professor, Internal Medicine, Division of General Medicine, Geriatrics and Palliative Care, University of Virginia Health System, Charlottesville, Virginia, United States

Mudhasir Bashir, MD
Associate Professor, Department of Psychiatry and Neurobehavioral Sciences, University of Virginia Health System, Charlottesville, Virginia

Oluwatoyin Falusi Nwafor, MD
Professor, Internal Medicine, Division of Infectious Diseases, Rush University Medical Center, Chicago, Illinois

Alwin Jeyakumar, MBBS
Professor, Internal Medicine, Division of Medical Oncology, Dalhousie University, Halifax, Nova Scotia, Canada

Moustafa Massoud, MD
Physician, Department of Internal Medicine, University of Alabama at Birmingham, Birmingham, Alabama.

Omar Massoud, MD, PhD
Chief, Hepatology Section, Department of Gastroenterology and Hepatology, Cleveland Clinic Foundation, Cleveland, Ohio.

Sula Mazimba, MD, MPH
Assistant Professor of Medicine, Division of Cardiovascular Medicine, University of Virginia
Charlottesville, Virginia.

Hunter Mwansa, MD
Department of Internal Medicine, OSF Saint Francis Medical Center, University of Illinois College of Medicine, Peoria, Illinois.

Olufemi O. Ojewuyi, MBBS, FWACS, FMCS
Consultant Urological Surgeon, Department of Surgery, Osun State University Teaching Hospital, Osogbo, Osun state, Nigeria

Adenrele Adedeji Olajide, MBBS, FACP, FACR
Associate Professor, Internal Medicine, Division of Rheumatology, Marshall University School of Medicine, Huntington, West Virginia, United States.

Omolola Olajide, MBBS, FACE, FACP
Associate Professor, Internal Medicine, Section of Endocrinology, Marshall School of Medicine
Huntington, West Virginia, United States.

Akhtar Purvez, MD
Clinical Anesthesiologist, Pain and Spine Center of Charlottesville, Charlottesville, Virginia

Faruk Turgut, MD
Professor, Internal Medicine, Division of Nephrology, Tayfur Ata Sokmen Faculty of Medicine, Hatay Mustafa Kemal University, Serinyol/Antakya/Hatay, Turkey 31100

About the Editor

Seki A. Balogun, MBBS, FACP, AGSF
Associate Professor, Internal Medicine and Geriatric Medicine
University of Virginia Health System, Charlottesville, Virginia, USA

Seki A. Balogun, MBBS, FACP, AGSF is an Associate Professor of Medicine and academic geriatrician at the University of Virginia Health System (UVA), Charlottesville, Virginia, United States, where she currently serves as the Director of the Geriatric Medicine Fellowship Program and Medical Director of a continuing care retirement community. As a Nigerian-American with medical training in Nigeria and the United States, she has had the privilege of providing medical care for older patients over three decades, in both countries and has an astute awareness of the different health issues faced by older patients across racial groups and ethnicities.

She was inducted into the University of Virginia Academy of Distinguished Educators in 2006 and is the recipient of numerous academic teaching and clinical awards including University of Virginia School of Medicine Excellence in Teaching award, UVA Department of Medicine Outstanding Clinical Care Award, U.S. News and World Report Top Doctors in Virginia, and Top Geriatrician in Charlottesville, VA, Top

Doctors Magazine. She has authored many peer reviewed publications and is co-editor for the book, Chronic Kidney Disease: Signs/Symptoms, Management Options and Potential Complications. Nova Science Publishers, Inc. 2013.

Index

A

B

C

D

E

F

G

H

I

M

N

O

P

Q

R

S

T

U

V

W

Y